Social Work with Psychiatric Patients

Social Work with Psychiatric Patients

Barbara L. Hudson

First published 1982 by
THE MACMILLAN PRESS LTD
London and Basingstoke
Companies and representatives throughout the world

ISBN 0 333 26685 4 (hard cover)
ISBN 0 333 26686 2 (paper cover)

Typeset in Hong Kong by
ASCO TRADE TYPESETTING LTD

Printed in Hong Kong

To my parents, Lorentz and Lorna Gullachsen

Contents

viii *Contents*

Preface

This book is about people who come under the care of a psychiatrist and about practical ways of helping them and their families. I have not set out to write a psychiatry textbook, nor to review the important sociological and philosophical issues that have figured prominently in the literature of the social work profession in recent years.

One study in a British social services department concluded that the social workers' involvement with the mentally ill was minimal: 'On the whole, the impression was gained that the social workers were holding a watching brief unless a crisis forced them to arrange the care of children or admission to hospital of adult clients' (Goldberg and Warburton, 1979). Other commentators are more critical: 'The social work role in relation to the mentally ill client has in most local authorities become stagnant, and the emphasis has remained upon outdated methods of intervention which has led to the atrophy of skill development' (Goldberg and Huxley, 1980). The low priority given to this client group may be related not only to shortage of resources but also to lack of specialised knowledge. This book is an attempt to go some way towards remedying this lack, and to offer suggestions for further study of mental disorder and how sufferers might be helped.

Several chapters focus on specific (and not so specific) diagnoses of mainstream psychiatry. Some social workers may find this objectionable. But an understanding of the language of psychiatry – how psychiatrists use terms like 'schizophrenia' or 'dementia' – is a *sine qua non* for mutually intelligible communication; and, moreover, research findings concerning some at least of the diagnostic groups do offer guidelines – working hypotheses – as to how we might begin to assist the individual and those around him. Several common disorders are described, 'from the outside', as it were; an attempt is made to convey something of the patient's and the family's experience; and common treatment approaches are outlined. I seek to draw conclusions about possible social work intervention from two main sources: from accounts and evaluations of treatment; and from the knowledge we have about psycho-social factors implicated in the course of each disorder – factors that may increase the likelihood of relapse, contribute to distress and disability, or intensify the burden on the family. Care is taken to distinguish between statements based only on experience and unsystematic observation, and statements based on empirical research. While my emphasis is on the latter, there are many areas where little is known, and others where what is known does not lead one to regard social work as having a major role in the helping process. For these reasons, the length of the sections is uneven – some topics get many pages, others a few lines. The chapters are not intended to be read in isolation: much of what is said about intervention in relation to one condition can apply to others.

The second part of the book deals with some general issues: the children of the psychiatric patient; accommodation, work and money problems; and aspects of social work in emergency situations and in the hospital setting.

If one can conceptualise mental disorder as a continuum ranging from the mild to the severe, then it is the severe end that is highlighted. Among many omissions, the reader will note that I have not covered child psychiatry, mental handicap or forensic psychiatry, and have mentioned only in passing special settings such as the therapeutic community and problems such as sexual dysfunction and marital discord, which often come to the attention of psychiatrists but do not in themselves constitute mental disorder. Each of these topics has its own specialist literature, whereas the literature of 'bread-and-butter' psychiatric social work is sparse.

There is a bias towards behavioural approaches. Apart from the fact that my own reading of the evidence suggests that this is a fruitful area in which social work can develop, I feel that this emphasis is justified on the grounds that psychodynamic approaches are adequately covered in other social work textbooks and that most social workers are already equipped to apply them when it seems appropriate to do so.

A central problem in writing this book has been how to depict the typical social worker. I cannot pretend to have solved it. I have drawn on personal experience and the descriptions of social work with psychiatric patients given in several research reports. The resulting composite picture is immodest, to say the least. My prototype possesses a wide range of skills and knowledge; he can do casework and groupwork according to a variety of different models; he is an administrator and a planner; he is a political campaigner; and his education has prepared him to read critically, to be articulate, and to be able to conceptualise his work and generalise appropriately from his experience. He is knowledgeable about psychology, sociology and social policy. And in addition to all this, I am suggesting that he can develop specialised skills for work in the psychiatric services!

I am aware that many, if not all of, the roles I suggest can be and are filled by other professional workers. The new profession of community psychiatric nursing has already added to basic nursing skills and knowledge much of the expertise that social work has traditionally considered to be its own province. Community psychiatry and community psychology have moved in a similar direction. Some observers have suggested that social work is being replaced with regard to the care of the mentally disordered in Britain; but, at the same time, there seems to be a renewed interest among social workers in this client group and in further training courses teaching specialist skills. In the USA, on the other hand, social workers appear to be undertaking a variety of innovative and responsible roles in the psychiatric services.

It is impossible to guess how far such trends are likely to go. The main purpose of this book is to help social workers with the task of applying their generic skills to the special problems of the mentally disordered in co-operation with other workers in the psychiatric services, and I believe this will continue to be important in the foreseeable future.

University of Oxford   BARBARA L. HUDSON

Acknowledgements

Jane Stainer read the whole manuscript. Individual chapters were read by Biddy Andrew, Vera Baraniecka, Rosemary Fitzgerald, Monica Greenwood, Roger McAuley, Pauline McDonnell, David Millard, Rolf Olsen, Brian Sheldon, Richard Stern and Kathy Sylva. They all helped me a great deal, and I am extremely grateful. Any errors, omissions and biases that remain are my own.

Brenda Dry typed and retyped with extraordinary patience and skill.

Steven Kennedy of the Macmillan Press Ltd provided effective reinforcement, both positive and negative.

B. L. H.

1

Introduction: Psychiatry and Social Work – Contention and Co-operation

Little if anything that the helping professions do for their patients and clients takes place outside a context of the values, rules, opportunities and constraints of the contemporary social system. This is nowhere more evident than in the field of psychiatry, and any mental health worker who is unaware of it is potentially dangerous. Social workers do not of course have a monopoly of sensitivity to social and ethical issues, of healthy scepticism about the medicalisation of problems of living, or of concern as to whether psychiatric intervention may not sometimes be more noxious than what it seeks to cure. But it does seem that social workers bring to their work a special awareness of these issues, which can do much to enrich or temper the deliberations of all those who are professionally involved with the individual who is described as 'mentally disordered', and this client group as a whole. This introductory chapter begins with an overview of some key issues which often arise as opposite sides in a pro- versus anti-psychiatry debate. However, mental disorder and its treatment is too multifaceted a topic for black-and-white notions.

At the centre of the debate are two main questions: (1) Is it harmful to be classified as 'mentally ill'? (2) Is it logical to use the term 'mental illness'? The sociological literature on labelling (for example, Scheff, 1974) highlights the importance of societal reaction to deviant behaviour. Certain people are designated 'mentally ill' by those whom society has authorised to do so, or by other people who can find no better explanation for their deviant behaviour. They may then react by producing more 'illness behaviour'. They may feel stigmatised and see themselves as second-class citizens and withdraw from others, or occasionally try to fight back; and whatever true disability they may have will interact with the negative expectations of others to produce further disability. They may become chronic 'patients' inside or outside hospital. Even if this does not happen, a record of psychiatric treatment and especially of involuntary hospitalisation can lead to a permanent change of status, with problems arising not only in informal relationships with other people but also in such areas as employment, emigration and relations with the legal system.

Further, the use of the term 'mental illness' can deter not only the patient, but also the family and society at large from taking responsibility for helping in treatment and rehabilitation and for the prevention of psychiatric disorder: 'If it's an illness it's the doctors' job.' Alcoholism provides an illustration of this problem. The notion that this is a disease can encourage the belief that individual effort has no part to play, and that social measures to limit alcohol consumption are irrelevant in the control of problem-drinking rates in the population. A diagnosis of 'depressive illness' can be taken as a signal to expect to be the passive recipient of pills or magic insights given out by a doctor; and the rest of society will regard proposals that social change might reduce the incidence of depression with considerable scepticism.

Some of these consequences of the 'mental illness' label relate to the logical issues surrounding the use of the term. This is to some extent, of course, a debate about the use of language. Does 'illness' mean the signs and symptoms of a known bodily dysfunction that can be treated by physical means, without reference to the person's beliefs and feelings, and to which his behaviour and his social environment are irrelevant? If that is what is implied, then many other 'illnesses' would have to be given another name. The vast range of physical disorders with causes and remedies that involve a complex interaction of psyche and soma and environment give the lie to any simplistic notion of what we mean by 'illness' and 'treatment'. We are being unfair to the general physician as well as to the psychiatrist if we assume that their so-called 'medical model' is a model of man as a machine with a mechanical fault, which can be mended by a technical expert who asks only that the machine be passive while he mends the broken part.

'Illness', then, is rarely a simple matter. It might be more valid to try to combat the notion held by patients, society and doctors alike that it is so, than to look for other language to describe the range of phenomena we now call 'mental illness'. The field of psychiatry encompasses a very wide variety of conditions, from the dementias with known physical damage to the brain, through schizophrenia with known hereditary as well as environmental components and suspected biochemical causes, to hysteria which mimicks physical malfunction without physical pathology. It is essential to recognise that mental illness is not a unitary phenomenon. There are degrees of potential self-help in its prevention and cure, degrees of environmental influence, and degrees of need for medical, psychological and social intervention. Not only does each diagnostic group differ from every other on all these dimensions, but each individual client or patient differs from every other. For some, the use of the term 'illness' can have benign effects: it can reduce feelings of guilt and anxiety for both the patient and his family. It allows care instead of control, or even punishment, for those whose behaviour has caused alarm or harm to other people. Although we usually wish to emphasise the need for partnership between client and helper, and the need for shared responsibility in putting matters right, we also want to put across a message of compassion. The attitude of the person concerned, and the nature of the disorder, interact to determine the most appropriate balance of responsibility to be placed on the client. Those who would want to insist that mental disorder is never 'illness', and would require everyone to take complete responsibility, should note where such extreme lines of argument can take us: Szasz (1974) describes schizophrenics as people who are inconsiderate of others, and recommends that their behaviour be controlled like that of other deviants, rather than 'treated', and all those who have suicidal impulses, he believes, should be allowed to 'take their lives' without interference.

Diagnosis is another form of labelling. Diagnosis in psychiatry is much less reliable than in other branches of medicine. Temerlin (1968) has demonstrated how readily psychiatrists can be swayed by suggestion, to the extent of diagnosing sanity or mental illness depending on how the 'patient' is presented to them. Rosenhan (1973) and seven volunteers were admitted to mental hospitals and complained only of one symptom: hearing voices saying 'thud' and 'hollow' and 'empty'. All were admitted. Although they then ceased to complain of their 'symptoms', all but one were diagnosed as schizophrenic. Upon release, the seven were described as 'schizophrenic in remission'. These experiments and others like them have no doubt contributed to the vigour with which the goal of more reliable diagnostic practices has been pursued in recent years, and there are certainly still no grounds for complacency.

But as Wing (1978) points out, bad practice does not invalidate the practice itself. Wing and his co-workers have demonstrated that diagnostic practice can be improved. Clare (1976) also argues that abuse of psychiatry in both the East and the West is facilitated by loose and unreliable diagnostic systems, and is less likely when psychiatrists are obliged to follow strict criteria for the recognition of mental disorder and the classification of the various syndromes.

Some diagnostic labels, however, remain little more than subjective comments by a psychiatrist: for example, 'psychopath' often means 'no other diagnoses fits (but I've got to classify him somehow)' and 'I don't like him' and 'I can't help him'. 'Psychopath' is, in addition, an example of a stigmatising label, which can colour the perceptions of all who get to know of it. In this case the stigma is more severe in psychiatrically 'sophisticated' circles. On the other hand, a diagnosis of schizophrenia is more disturbing to the lay person, as a result of public ignorance and bad publicity: it conjures up images of Dr Jekyll and Mr Hyde (the mistaken notion of schizophrenia as split personality), or of the very rare cases of violence that are widely reported in the newspapers.

Diagnosis can also have the effect of de-individualising – invalidating – the person who is diagnosed; all his qualities, except those that are subsumed under the diagnostic label, may be disregarded. Attempts to avoid this have led to the introduction of such terms as 'the person with schizophrenia' instead of 'the schizophrenic' in order to stress that this person is in very many respects like no other person and in very many respects like all other people. Social workers make a valuable contribution in emphasising the individual and the universal; doctors risk concerning themselves too narrowly with the diagnostic category. While narrowness of view is a danger in all branches of medicine (for example, on maternity wards) it is of particular importance for psychiatric patients who are especially vulnerable to feeling devalued. If the person is living in an institution and depends very heavily on professional workers for his sense of worth, the hurt will be even more pronounced.

A further problem with diagnostic labels is that they can lead to inappropriate and possibly damaging generalisations, and to premature decisions about the person's prognosis and ability to respond which may turn into self-fulfilling prophecies. The person with senile dementia may be deprived of stimulation, medical care, ordinary respect. The psychopath is assumed to be always 'manipulative' and never depressed, and is denied even the assistance that the rest of our clients can expect from the social and medical services. The schizophrenic is no longer listened to, and his abilities and strengths are forgotten.

Once again, these are examples of bad practice, rather than inevitable consequences of diagnosis. Watson (1979) argues that diagnostic enthusiasts are less often guilty of de-individualising psychiatric patients than are the sociologists who write of mental illness as if it were a unitary concept, and the anti-diagnosis workers in settings such as the therapeutic community, where all the patients are often treated alike regardless of diagnosis. Even writers who have drawn attention to the failings of psychiatry, such as Temerlin and Rosenhan, have not denied the possibility that there may exist clusters of symptoms that regularly occur together and have different causes and different cures, even if these have not to date been identified. A group of symptoms can turn out to have a particular organic basis (as in the case of general paralysis of the insane, now known to be caused by the syphilitic spirochaete), or to show a particular pattern of inheritance (for example, Huntington's Chorea), or to respond to a specific form of medication (for example, schizophrenia).

Knowledge advances by a process that begins with categorisation according to specific, repeatable observations; this is followed by the formation of hypotheses concerning the categories, and then the testing of the hypotheses. In other words, research is impossible without categorisation. This is as true of psychiatry as of any other field of study. For certain diagnostic groups, some compelling evidence about cause, course, and treatment has been obtained; the diagnostic categorisation has already proved its worth. In the chapters that follow there will be many examples of what has been achieved – for instance, the evidence concerning family relationships in schizophrenia and in depression, the effects of medication on these two major disorders, the effectiveness of behaviour therapy in the treatment of phobias. It is not possible, of course, to produce universal laws, only statements of probability. For example, it is probable that a certain kind of family interaction will be associated with relapse in schizophrenia; it is probable that a person who suffers recurrent attacks of hypomania will have fewer relapses if he receives lithium carbonate. Such statements of probability are of immense value in planning for the patients involved. Practice needs to be anchored in knowledge; the knowledge base of psychiatry is limited but it is growing. Although accumulated practice wisdom must not be devalued, it has to be supplemented and often supplanted by knowledge derived from meticulous research. Research has already provided generalisations that offer a good starting point in individual cases. This body of knowledge would not exist were it not for the efforts of workers who have focused on reliable diagnosis.

Despite these advances, there remains the argument that it is better not to fall into the hands of psychiatrists, not only because of their damaging labels and the harmful psychological and social processes that can be set in train, but for the straightforward reason that psychiatric patients are maltreated and unjustly deprived of freedom and human dignity, by psychiatrists themselves or by other staff in the psychiatric services, sometimes out of deliberate cruelty, more often through neglect, or well-meant but ignorant enthusiasm for the 'treatment' being given. Reports of the conditions in psychiatric hospitals, the results of public enquiries, and well-documented accounts of individual cases of mistreatment and injustice have highlighted the need for far stronger safeguards than are currently in operation. In order to stamp out abuses, much greater public awareness and sympathy need to be created; and the power of strong professions to protect their activities from outside scrutiny and debate, and their members from the consequences of malpractice, needs to be curtailed. Large institutions, isolated from the rest of society, need to be opened to the outside world, or, better still, abolished altogether.

However, the abolition of psychiatry itself is hardly likely to bring an end to the ill-treatment of those whom we describe as mentally ill; history, and an examination of the practices in countries where psychiatry is less influential, provide clear evidence of this. The author remembers hearing about a madwoman led by a rope, amid jeers from her neighbours, in a remote part of Europe; such scenes were not uncommon in nineteenth-century Britain. History provides numerous instances of the cruelty that can result if mental illness does not figure in explanations of bizarre or deviant behaviour. It is true that these evils did not disappear when asylums replaced prisons and workhouses, and doctors and nurses replaced witch-finders and gaolers. The asylums came to resemble the prisons, and some of the 'treatments' were little better than chains or outright assault. However, the cruelties of psychiatry, and its harmful 'treatments', and the continuing indifference or worse of the public at large, are not a function of psychiatry and the psychiatric services *per se*: they are due to ignorance, insensitivity, or lack of resources, and they implicate not only the medical services but the society that employs them. Many of the real advances that have occurred over the last thirty years owe much to enlightened doctors and to medical researchers. The drugs that maintain so many patients in the community who would otherwise be kept in institutions, and the physical treatments that bring the severely depressed back into contact with their world, are the inventions of psychiatrists. Looking back further, it was Pinel, a physician, who insisted on unchaining the Bicêtre Asylum inmates, and Connolly, also a physician, who introduced 'moral treatment' at Hanwell Asylum.

It is mischievous to equate bad hospitals and bad treatment with the institution of psychiatry. Attacks have to be aimed at those who are guilty of malpractice and the systems that shield them from outside scrutiny, and not indiscriminately.

It is unfortunate, both for the relationship between the professions, and also for the fate of the mentally disordered patient or client, that so many social workers have been influenced by one side only in the anti-psychiatry debate. Psychiatrists such as Wing (1978), Clare (1976) and Eisenberg (1977) have considered these issues without hysterical counter-attack and without denying the abuses that exist. Social workers need to become more aware of the achievements of modern psychiatry, and, without becoming uncritical psychiatrists' aides, they need to work alongside them in order to achieve more humane and better services.

As research continues and empirical data accumulate, some questions that at present are matters of ideology become questions of fact. For example, the long-term consequences of being labelled 'mentally disordered' are being assessed (for a brief review of the somewhat equivocal findings to date, see Fitzgerald, 1982). The feasibility of shorter hospital stays, and the possibility of overcoming the obstacles to returning to work, are being methodically explored (Hirsch *et al.*, 1979; Wansbrough and Cooper, 1980). And, as mentioned earlier, the fact that diagnostic reliability can be improved, and the value of grouping psychiatric symptoms under diagnoses, are being demonstrated for several diagnostic categories. In so far as empirically based knowledge is absorbed by both social workers and psychiatrists, so the two groups will find it easier to join together in a productive working relationship. Value questions will remain, of course, and social workers will continue to ask them (so will many doctors, psychologists and nurses). But at the same time, we have to accept that if we are to have the maximum opportunity to bring our skills to the people who need them, we have to work alongside the medical profession: psychiatrists are entrusted with the major responsibility for those whom society calls mentally ill, and their authority is accepted by patients and their families. We need to be able to communicate and fit in with the rest of the team. This does not, of course, mean that we should become obedient technicians, carrying out orders without reference to the intangible but real and far-reaching issues of human rights and dignity.

The concept of teamwork in psychiatry is a problematic one – and the problems are certainly not all of the social worker's making! Teamwork does not mean a single thinker and decision-maker with a staff of subordinates to do his bidding (a view held, it would appear, by a number of consultant psychiatrists). It is a group of professionals who share in assessment, planning and treatment, co-operating to provide a comprehensive and well co-ordinated service. Each member contributes according to his skills and the client's or family's needs, and the contribution of each will vary from case to case. The recipients of the service do not feel confused or embarrassed at the variety of professionals intervening in their lives, but reassured that a group of people will help them in variety of ways.

A number of research studies have shown us a rather different reality: lack of mutual respect, power struggles, poor co-ordination, and some members – especially social workers, but often also nurses and psychologists – feeling undervalued and under-used (Hunt, 1979; Miles, 1977; Sanson-Fisher *et al.*, 1979). Patients who have been persuaded to appear before a roomful of strangers at a case conference may be justified in feeling that this is an audience rather than a team of helpers, and they are often given the message that unless a doctor is seeing them they are being fobbed off with second-best.

It would be fanciful to suggest that with more goodwill, status rivalry and bad teamwork will just go away. It is important that members of the team clarify their potential contributions for one another, and learn about each other's background knowledge and range of skills. This cannot be a once-and-for-all exercise, since individual workers add to their competencies and sometimes change direction over time. Generally speaking, there are areas of exclusive competence, such as pharmacotherapy or psychological testing; areas of exclusive responsibility, such as duties under the mental-health or child-protection legislation; and areas of overlap, such as psychotherapy, groupwork, family therapy, behaviour therapy. We should acknowledge that some members of a profession may lack skills usually expected of that profession: some psychiatrists (in Britain, perhaps most) have had no training in psychotherapy, and there are some psychologists who have not trained in behaviour therapy. On the other hand, some members of professions have skills not usually associated with those professions; some nurses are highly skilled in behaviour therapy; some occupational therapists have trained in group therapy. The social worker is often the best qualified person to undertake family therapy and other forms of 'talking treatment'.

Social workers are the least predictable occupational group with regard to what they are able to offer, and have – perhaps deservedly – been much criticised on this account. Generally speaking, their particular spheres of interest are the social factors that exacerbate the plight of people with mental disorder, such as poverty, unemployment and poor housing, interpersonal relationships, and the welfare of the family as a whole. They tend to have a good knowledge of social norms, and, as we noted earlier, an awareness of the dangers inherent in entry into the 'sick role' and of the negative consequences of psychiatric intervention. However, the range of skill and knowledge to be found within social work is extremely wide. Some social workers offer treatment that is scarcely distinguishable from psychotherapy; others specialise in welfare rights; in the USA, social workers can be found in charge of a community crisis intervention centre or a behavioural in-patient treatment ward. Because of the bewildering array of possible competencies it is essential that other professionals do not have to try to co-operate with a large number of unfamiliar social workers, who are prevented by their allegiance to a different agency from taking a full part in the psychiatric service. As the social worker becomes known to the rest of the team, so the requests made to him will become more appropriate to his skills; at the same time, he will become better able to respond to the requirements of the team's clientele.

The social worker can play a useful role at all stages of psychiatric care: diagnosis, treatment and rehabilitation. Diagnosis is traditionally a closely guarded prerogative of the medically qualified, and certainly the psychiatrist's training in this part of the work is unlikely to be surpassed by that of any other profession. The British Association of Social Workers Working Party (1974) suggests that social workers can contribute on two levels: (a) screening as to need for a psychiatric opinion, and (b) contribution to psychiatric diagnosis, and use of psychiatric knowledge in social assessment. For the screening task the social worker needs to be familiar with the kinds of behaviour and complaints that are considered in making a psychiatric diagnosis. For the second and more specialised level of contribution, he needs knowledge and experience of particular symptoms and the sense that is likely to be made of them by a psychiatrist. Although perhaps beyond the call of duty, the specialist knowledge that some social workers possess can have far-reaching results. An example of this was a probation officer's report on a client who had been detained in a mental hospital following a minor assault. This report, without suggesting a formal diagnosis, commented on the absence of various symptoms that might have attracted a diagnosis of severe mental illness. The probation officer also noted the client's lack of fluency in English, his intense anxiety, and his fear of 'the authorities', and linked these to his status as a recent immigrant. She went on to mention that his conversation, although disjointed, was not muddled; his beliefs fitted in with his cultural background, and his history and current life-style were typical of his subculture; he was not confused, and he had coped satisfactorily with work and social relationships in the past. In this case the probation officer's report helped the defence psychiatrist to exclude the possibility of mental illness, whereas previous psychiatrists without her report had given the man a diagnosis of paranoid schizophrenia. The author, on interviewing a woman complaining of sexual problems, elicited information that suggested that she was suffering from a 'classical' depressive illness. On referral to a psychiatrist this was confirmed, and she responded rapidly to treatment for the depression, and had no need of sex therapy.

Systematic evidence of the potential of social workers in assessment (very heartening at a time when doubt is being cast on our competence from so many quarters!) is given by Newson-Smith and Hirsch (1979), whose research on the assessment of overdose patients demonstrated that the social workers in the study were at least as good at detecting illness as the psychiatrists.

The social worker's varying contributions to treatment and re-habilitation, as well as to assessment and diagnosis, are discussed in the ensuing chapters. The greater the social worker's sophistication in psychiatry, the more he can contribute. And this is no sell-out to the so-called medical model – this kind of sophistication can coexist with the generic principles, knowledge and methods that basic social work training has provided.

Part 1
Psychiatric Disorders

2

Schizophrenia

The doctors in Rosenhan's (1973) experiment diagnosed schizophrenia solely on the basis of a complaint of hearing voices, and in the Soviet Union dissidents can be labelled schizophrenic on the grounds that they hold deviant political beliefs. In modern British psychiatry, on the other hand, schizophrenia is narrowly defined. The clarification of differences in diagnostic practice at different places, and the development of clear-cut and reliable criteria, have had significant consequences, facilitating the replication of research studies and the interpretation of their results, and helping us to make sense of the bewildering array of expositions of aetiology and treatment in the literature. Where a wider, less exclusive system is used, many people are labelled schizophrenic who would be considered to have an affective psychosis, a neurotic disorder, or a personality disorder, under the stricter system. In this book, the term 'schizophrenia' is used only in the strict sense.

The key symptoms (known as 'first-rank symptoms,' originally described by Kurt Schneider) include:

(a) *feelings of passivity*, that is, the experience that one's thoughts or actions are under external control
(b) *auditory hallucinations* in the form of more than one voice talking *about* the patient *in the third person*
(c) *primary delusions*, that is, the experience in which the person suddenly becomes convinced that a particular set of events has a special meaning (this conviction is out of keeping with beliefs held by other people in the same social or cultural group).

Other frequently occurring symptoms are auditory hallucinations in which a voice or voices are talking *to* the patient, at times calling him names and abusing him, or giving him orders. In addition there

is a subjective difficulty in thinking, with bizarre connections between thoughts, and apparent blocks in the stream of thought. Many
patients build up a complex delusional system comprising a network
of ideas, often bizarre but all interrelated, which serve to explain the
reason for the original delusion or the auditory hallucinations.

Several of these symptoms are found in other types of mental
illness. For example, severely depressed people may suffer from
delusions, and are then said to be suffering from 'psychotic
depression'.

Chronic schizophrenia can bring about a breakdown in the individual's social skills, and severe social withdrawal. There may be
flatness of emotional expression ('flatness of affect'), or a tendency
to laugh on sad occasions ('incongruity of affect'). A person suffering
from chronic schizophrenia is apathetic, slow in thoughts and movements, and tends to neglect his dress and at times his personal
hygiene.

The prognosis in schizophrenia is variable. After a first acute
episode, about a third of the patients recover completely. This group
comprises mainly those without a family history of schizophrenia,
and with an obvious precipitating 'life event', and their illness is
characterised by sudden onset, depression, and the absence of
apathy. Prompt treatment is an important factor in a satisfactory
outcome. Others suffer further acute relapses, but between these
episodes they recover to some extent, though with some deterioration in their work and social abilities. The indicators of poor prognosis are a family history of schizophrenia and a slow insidious
onset (usually during the teens or early twenties). Up to one-third of
patients do not recover, except from some of the florid symptoms,
and spend the rest of their lives suffering severe handicap. Their
difficulties are often exacerbated by additional neurotic symptoms,
such as anxiety, depression and obsessions.

Because more psychiatric patients are handicapped by schizophrenia than by any other condition, except the organic disorders of
old age, and because schizophrenia resembles prototypical images
of 'insanity', there has been more research and speculation about
this illness than any other form of mental disorder. It has been at the
centre of ideological controversy, and has preoccupied all schools of
investigator, from the psychoanalyst to the biochemist. Few theories
of causation have much hard evidence to support them, and some,

such as the theories of existential or political reaction, have no research support whatsoever.

However, recent investigations of the brain biochemistry and psychophysiology of schizophrenia are beginning to yield results (Iversen, 1978; Venables, 1979). There is also strong evidence of an hereditary component, perhaps inheritance of vulnerability to the development of schizophrenia. However, of those with a close relative who develops schizophrenia, only one person in ten will himself develop the disorder (Office of Health Economics, 1979). Leff (1978) sums up the current state of knowledge as follows:

> The work discussed ... has suggested that the contribution of genes to the eventual development of 'schizophrenia' is approximately 50 per cent. Whatever the size of the proportion, it is clear that environmental factors play a substantial part in aetiology. Some of them ... are likely to be somatic in nature. Others are psychological or social.

The best-known theories concerning environmental causes of schizophrenia are those of Bateson *et al.* (1956) (the 'double-bind'), Lidz *et al.* (1965) ('marital skew' and 'marital schism'), Wynne *et al.* (1958) ('pseudo-mutuality') and Laing and Esterson (1964) ('conspiratorial').

Research on the 'family causation hypothesis' has failed to confirm the theories of these writers, whose views seem to have had an undeserved influence on their social work readership. After a thorough review of this research, Hirsch and Leff (1975) conclude that only a few general statements can be made with any degree of confidence: (a) parents of schizophrenics are more often psychiatrically disturbed than parents of normal children, (b) there is a link between allusive thinking (i.e. over-generalised, irrelevant speech) in schizophrenics and their parents, but this is also true of normal people and their parents, though rarer in them; (c) parents of schizophrenics show more conflict than parents of other patients, (d) people who later develop schizophrenia suffer more illness as children than the rest of the population; (e) mothers of people who later develop schizophrenia show more 'overconcern' than parents, of other children; (f) some careful but unconfirmed research (Singer and Wynne, 1965) suggests that the parents of schizophrenics may have abnormal speech patterns. All these findings can be explained in terms of a common heredity shared by both parents and children, or by reference to the observation that cause-and-effect can work in the opposite direction: the ill health or oddness of the child might be affecting the parent.

It is important for social workers to take note of this and other rigorous examinations of the evidence, because much bad publicity has accrued to the parents of schizophrenic patients, who already suffer an immense enough burden without being made to feel responsible for the patient's illness.

What does it feel like? It is extremely difficult to imagine the experience of being psychotic; indeed a sense of remoteness, of not being able to reach the patient, is often used as data to support the diagnosis. Perhaps the closest we can get is to recall our nightmares, and the feeling of dread engendered quite irrationally by certain culturally determined sets of circumstances: the footsteps behind us on a dark night, the moving curtains, the creaking shutters in horror films. Add to this the feeling we all sometimes have of being 'hassled' by other people, and wishing they would leave us in peace. But this is perhaps as far as an attempt at empathy can take us. Indeed, it may be that to try too hard is not in anyone's best interests. For example, one patient responded to his social worker's comment that she partially understood how he felt by claiming that the social worker, like him, was 'different' – and that 'they' were out to get the social worker as well!

Priest (see Priest and Steinert, 1977) provides a helpful discussion of understandability. He takes a middle path between the view that the statements of thought-disordered patients are meaningless, and the view that they communicate matters of great significance and can be understood if one looks for symbols and connections. The latter may or may not be true and is difficult to verify; what is clear is that when drug treatment has lessened other symptoms, speech can return to normal. There is no reason to suppose that simple expressions of caring are any less valuable than more 'sophisticated' attempts to provide 'talking treatment'. Indeed the latter course might constitute further stress for the patient.

Accounts of what it feels like to suffer from schizophrenia have been published in *Schizophrenia from Within* (Wing, 1975). What comes across most vividly is the fear, suspicion and self-doubt, and the feeling that the world has somehow gone wrong. These descriptions are by people who have recovered from acute attacks. It is perhaps even more difficult to understand what it is like for the chronic schizophrenic patient. Priest (Priest and Steinert, 1977) points out that many suffer from anxiety and depression and are aware at some level of their difference from others. The National Schizophrenia Fellowship has published a series of descriptions by relatives: *Living with Schizophrenia* (1974a). The strain experienced by these families is enormous. Not only are they distressed – sometimes angered, sometimes frightened and sometimes bewildered – but they also suffer from a great deal of guilt and a feeling of helplessness, because they do not know how they ought to respond to the patient's behaviour. Further suffering results from deficiencies in the services: families are often treated like 'cases', considered to be over-anxious or over-involved, made to feel more guilty, kept in ignorance of the diagnosis and prognosis, and given little or no advice about how to cope. Ways in which social workers could assist the families are discussed later in this chapter.

Medical treatment

The drug group known as the phenothiazines, which are major tranquillisers, are the most usual and the most effective form of treatment for schizophrenia, in both its chronic and acute manifestations. These drugs do help to suppress florid symptoms and help the patient to cope outside hospital (Hirsch *et al.*, 1973; Leff and Wing, 1971).

However, there are a variety of side-effects, some of which can be severe. They may cause tremor and restlessness, curious postures, a blank expression and facial grimaces, protrusion of the tongue and chewing movements. Some of these side-effects may be lessened by administration of antiparkinsonian drugs. These can help to reduce stiffness and tremor, but some of the movements, such as protrusion of the tongue and chewing movements, may be permanent in some cases. They are particularly distressing because they make the person look odd, leading to further stigma. Recent research may soon provide psychiatrists with information as to how they may prevent these effects by more sophisticated prescribing, but at the present time psychiatrists need to be very sure of their diagnosis and the necessity of this treatment before they put patients on phenothiazines. This holds true despite the fact that some authorities consider that delay can be harmful (Clare, 1976; Priest and Woolfson, 1978). Social workers may be in a position to keep the medical staff informed of the occurrence of side-effects; we should note that sometimes a decrease in the amount of drug is not the answer, so that pleas to take the patient off his medication may be misguided.

Other fairly common side-effects include dry mouth, blurred vision, constipation, and failure of ejaculation. Some patients complain of drowsiness and gaining weight.

Many patients on phenothiazines are given them in the form of intramuscular 'depot' injections, which last from one to four weeks. Apart from ensuring that the patient does in fact receive the medication as prescribed, this system allows opportunity for regular contact with either the doctor or the psychiatric nurse.

There is disagreement among the various authorities as to how long treatment should continue, but most patients who have relapsed once can expect to receive the drug for a year or two at least.

Social factors

Despite their proven efficacy, the drugs do not always prevent relapse, neither do they influence the negative symptoms of schizophrenia, such as apathy and social withdrawal. During a trial of Modecate (a long-acting injectable phenothiazine), the sociologist in the research team found that 75 per cent of relatives of patients *not* on the drug complained of severe burden, but of relatives of patients who *were* on the drug, as many as 50 per cent also complained of severe burden (Stevens, 1973a). In the study by Vaughn and Leff (1976) it was shown that drugs did indeed protect patients from relapsing when under stress, but stress itself was of great significance. From these and other reports, it is clear that the success of out-patient maintenance depends on a very complex interaction between pharmacological and psycho-social aspects of care.

The environment can be harmful in three major respects: (1) over-stimulation, which increases the probability of relapse; (2) under-stimulation, which maintains or increases chronic disability; and, overlapping with (2), (3) people in the patient's environment can encourage maladaptive behaviour by reinforcing it, or discourage 'healthy' behaviour by failing to reinforce, or even by punishing it.

These mechanisms have been studied in considerable detail in a series of well-designed research programmes.

Overstimulation is perhaps the easiest to identify and the hardest to prevent, especially when the person is living outside the protective hospital environment. Overstimulation means being exposed to events or situations that arouse emotions or make excessive demands on the person's ability to cope. There is some evidence that schizophrenic patients may be more sensitive than other people, even when they appear severely withdrawn. They have been described by the psychophysiologist, Venables (1964), as being flooded with sensory impressions from all quarters. When they withdraw it may be to protect themselves.

The best-known example of overstimulation is the role of 'life events'. Patients who suffer onset or relapse of schizophrenia are more likely to have recently experienced a 'life event' in the previous three weeks than a control group of 'well' members of the general population (Brown and Birley, 1968). 'Life events' include obviously painful experiences, like the death of a relative or being made redundant, rather less obvious ones like losing a pet, and even events that might on the face of it seem very positive, such as being promoted or inheriting a large sum of money. Other research has shown that sudden placement in a new and demanding situation – for example, joining an industrial rehabilitation course – may have similar effects (Wing, Bennett and Denham, 1964).

Of particular interest to social workers are the findings concerning the 'high expressed emotion' home (Brown, Birley and Wing, 1972; Vaughn and Leff, 1976). The phrase 'high expressed emotion' refers to statements made by relatives indicating criticism, hostility or over-involvement towards the patient. Patients with relatives who were rated high on 'expressed emotion' had a much higher relapse rate than other schizophrenic patients, and critical comments were the most significant factor. But if the patient was not in their company full-time, if he was out at work or attending a day-centre, then he seemed to be protected by this. Medication also provided protection. The main conclusion, then, is that schizophrenic patients are more likely to relapse if they are not on drugs and spend a lot of time in the company of relatives who express a great deal of criticism towards them.

It seems reasonable to extrapolate from these findings to other aspects of the patient's experience. For example, one researcher found that schizophrenic patients disliked therapy groups at a day-hospital and did not take part in the discussions, and that some of them became disturbed, possibly as a consequence of the group (Stevens, 1973b). A social worker writing about her groupwork with schizophrenic patients describes their need for a very stable setting – even a change of therapy room upset them, and they tended to withdraw if the discussion became too personal or emotional (Sheppard, 1960). These observations fit in with the results of the research outlined above.

The converse of overstimulation also has serious consequences for the schizophrenic patient. Understimulation is a major factor in institutionalisation. Social withdrawal, 'flatness of affect', and poverty of speech are all greatly influenced by the kind of environment the patient lives in, and the most important aspect is how much there is for the patient to do. Another key factor is the attitude of the staff with regard to the person's potential for improvement. Unfortunately, leaving hospital does not automatically solve the problem. Hostels can be as understimulating as hospitals (Apte, 1968), and many patients living at home spend a great deal of their time doing nothing (Brown *et al.*, 1966; Stevens, 1972).

Finally, there is the related problem of the people around the patient placing him firmly in the sick-role. This attitude shows itself in the 'does he take sugar?' phenomenon; low expectations; and rewards for abnormal behaviour such as delusional talk or lying in bed all day rather than rewards for acting normally. Hospital studies (for example, Ayllon and Azrin, 1968) have shown that nurses' choice of which type of behaviour to attend to and which to ignore has a powerful influence on the 'normality' or otherwise of the people in their care. What is true of nurses is almost certainly true of anyone else who interacts regularly with the patient.

The social worker's role

Clearly, with a condition as complex as schizophrenia, a multidisciplinary approach is essential. Some of the social work roles may overlap with those of colleagues in other professions.

First a social history is needed including details of the patient's personal relationships and work experience, and of his life-style prior to onset of his illness; this information will assist the psychiatrist in confirming his diagnosis and may provide pointers with regard to prognosis. In planning the drug treatment and future care, such as day-hospital attendance, the team will value information about the person's current and expected environment. An account of how he spends his day, the quality and amount of interaction with the family, even details about the house – whether the patient can get privacy and peace – constitute important information. Later on, observations about drug effects should also be reported. In this connection it is worth noting that certain side-effects, such as the oculogyric crisis, where there is a spasm of the muscles, causing the eyes to turn upwards, may be interpreted by the family as just another piece of attention-seeking or bizarre behaviour, and not reported. Similarly, restlessness and inability to sit still may be taken to be a sign of anxiety or boredom.

Apart from 'reporting back', the social worker has a wide choice of possible intervention strategies to help the patient and the family. If we consider the three groups of psycho-social factors it is clear that there is a considerable role for social work.

Our knowledge of the ill effects of understimulation suggests that a major task is to try to prevent inactivity. Clearly the most straight-forward preventive action is to ensure that the patient does not become institutionalised in hospital or elsewhere. This may mean referral to a day-centre, help with accommodation and work on leaving hospital, or asking the consultant to keep a place in the hospital's industrial or occupational therapy programme for those patients whose life at home is known to be understimulating. Help from volunteers, voluntary associations, and friends and relatives of the patient, can be marshalled, to improve the opportunities for interesting and constructive activity. Some patients have special interests that can be encouraged: for example, chronic schizophrenic patients known to the author have enjoyed playing bridge and chess, helping in a neighbour's garden, and in one large hostel for home-less men were given 'special' jobs to do. In tackling the problem of understimulation, and indeed other difficulties in this client group, we should note that the traditional casework approach, where the client is guided to find his own solutions at his own speed, is unlikely to be helpful for the chronic schizophrenic patient, whose apathy and tendency to withdraw require a more directive style on the social worker's part.

The problem of overstimulation seems to demand a protective

style of working. Notions about learning the hard way, and of the potential for change at times of crisis, have no place in casework with the schizophrenic patient. As we have noted, any change of life-style, such as a return to work, or a move from one living environment to another, needs to be carefully prepared for and accomplished gradually. These clients will require help with many day-to-day problems, of a kind we might encourage others to deal with for themselves: legal, housing or financial problems. A balance must be struck between being paternalistic and expecting too much of the client.

While it is important not to assume that most families are 'high expressed emotion' families (Vaughn and Leff (1976) found this situation in only about one-third, and of course the family atmosphere may vary over time), when such a situation has been recognised we have to try to protect the patient from stressful interaction. A variety of strategies are possible. Encouraging the relatives and patient to spend more time apart might be achieved by finding occupation for either the patient *or* the relative outside the home. In some homes it may be important to try to obtain more privacy for the patient.

A more ambitious goal is to try to modify the family interaction directly. The social worker with skills in behaviour therapy might use the communication training approach (see, for example, Thomas, 1977), with the family as a group, or possibly the key relatives on their own. This would require particular care to avoid placing stress on the clients. A more traditional social work approach is to encourage the relatives to talk about their feelings to the worker. This might have the effect of diverting the expression of emotion away from the patient. It is probably the most-used style of work at the present time, but there are major theoretical objections to it. There is little evidence to suggest that 'ventilation' has anything but a short-term tension-releasing effect; and further, there is some evidence that it simply leads to expressing more hostility (Saunders, 1977). If, however, the relatives can come to a better understanding of the patient and their own reactions to him, then they might be able to gain greater control over their own behaviour. It is certainly important for the relatives to feel that they are understood and accepted, and that they receive the recognition they deserve for the burden they carry in continuing to provide the patient with a home. Needless to say, they should not be given the impression that the worker thinks they caused the disorder.

Relatives' groups can indirectly affect family interaction, and have numerous other useful functions (Priestley, 1979). Relatives themselves can provide much helpful advice on how to cope with irritating behaviour on the patient's part. Here are some suggestions reported by Creer and Wing (1974): instead of nagging the patient to change his clothes, just put out a set of clean ones; look the other way when he displays unpleasant table manners; make a friendly agreement as to where he can talk about his delusions; receive delusional talk in a neutral way, neither encouraging nor condemning it. (Professionals as well as other relatives can learn a great deal from the many families of schizophrenics who have become considerably more competent in providing a caring and helpful environment than many paid helpers would be.)

Berkowitz, Kuipers and Leff (1981) have recently reported the results of a combined intervention programme for patients and relatives in the 'high expressed emotion' group. In addition to medication, the programme has three elements: education, a family interview, and a fortnightly relatives' group. The relatives receive teaching sessions on the diagnosis, symptoms, causes, treatment and management of schizophrenia. In the family interview, ways of reducing contact are discussed and an attempt is made to resolve family conflicts. The groups are run as self-help groups, with the staff acting as facilitators. Relatives from 'low expressed emotion' homes join in the sessions, and the members discuss coping strategies and provide mutual support and information. The results are very encouraging indeed: although the amount of contact between relatives and patients has proved difficult to alter, many of the relatives have reduced their level of 'expressed emotion'; and relapse rates have decreased. Although one must always be cautious about basing practice on the results of a single study, it does seem that work along these lines is likely to be a preferred form of service for this client group in the future.

Another approach to problems of family interaction, as well as to the rehabilitation of the chronic schizophrenic patient, is to try to identify which of the patient's behaviours cause most distress or annoyance to others, and to seek to modify these with or without setting up a full-scale family behaviour modification programme. Projects of this kind have been described by Cheek *et al.* (1971a), Hudson (1975a) and Atkinson (1977). Similar work on hospital wards has proved very effective (see, for example, Stöffelmayr *et al.*, 1973), but this is a difficult undertaking in the home setting. Also, it seems that if the patient has florid symptoms, or is unresponsive to social reinforcement, behavioural approaches are unlikely to succeed. This said, there will be some cases for which a behavioural programme on operant-conditioning lines is well worth trying. Preferably, the family are brought in as co-therapists along with the worker. Behavioural deficits, such as failure to help with household chores, or problem behaviour, such as constantly talking about delusions, are carefully specified, and an attempt is made to shape up more acceptable patterns of behaviour by consistently rewarding any slight improvement, while ignoring unwanted behaviour. Behavioural workers have also begun to develop social skills training in groups for chronic schizophrenic patients, and the results are promising (Bellack and Hersen, 1979). The social worker using these approaches has to take care not to expect too much too soon, and to avoid making the patient feel he is under too close scrutiny or, worse, under attack.

One potential source of stress is the social worker himself and the methods he employs. Schizophrenic clients should not be subjected to the rigours of insight-giving or confrontative casework and groupwork. Plenty of support should be provided, along with gentle encouragement to stay with reality, to put psychotic material to the back of his mind and dismiss strange thoughts. Sometimes we can offer face-saving methods of coping with the knowledge that one is 'different', while at the same time accepting the need for special help. These patients should be spared the experience of having to get to know a variety of workers; they require regular long-term contact with one person whom they can learn to trust and who does not make emotional demands. This means that the agency should try to allocate a worker who is likely to remain in post for some time – these clients need to be classed along with children in care, as requiring special consideration in this respect.

This chapter has concentrated on working with individuals and families. With the growing emphasis on community care for this group, and a small increase in optimism about their future in the community, there has been a steady flow of research literature on the development of services outside hospital. The topics of employment, accommodation and financial provision are taken up in more detail in Chapters 11 and 12, and they need to be considered alongside attempts to help with living skills and personal relationships.

3

Hypomania and Severe Depressive Illness (The Affective Psychoses)

Hypomania and severe depressive illness are called 'affective' disorders because the key feature is abnormal mood. 'Psychosis' indicates a severe form of mental disorder; hypomania has in common with schizophrenia a resemblance to the layman's notion of insanity, at least during the acute phase, and some manifestations of depressive illness also have this quality. Nevertheless, complete recovery is usual, although there may be frequent relapses.

These two disorders can sometimes alternate in the same individual (manic-depressive psychosis). Hypomania is much rarer than depression.

Hypomania

'Intense well-being ... restrictions or confinement are apt at times to produce extreme irritation and even paroxysms of anger' – thus writes an ex-patient of his experience of mania (Custance, 1952). Mania is the severe form of this disorder, nowadays usually forestalled by early medical treatment. Hypomania is the milder form which is more often seen.

The hypomanic patient may appear superficially to be in extra high spirits: energetic, cheerful, optimistic, a little boastful and overbearing, perhaps. But on closer acquaintance he is seen to be overactive, grandiose, often irritable, and occasionally aggressive towards anyone who puts obstacles in his way. He may have delusions, especially of grandeur. He is egocentric, insensitive to other people, often meddlesome, and he seems oblivious to the moral scruples he normally holds. His speech becomes rapid and rambling, with flight of ideas (jumping from topic to topic). One of the most alarming features is his impulsive behaviour, such as running up large debts, resigning his job, quarrelling with friends and colleagues, or walking out on his family. Sometimes the problems are compounded by heavy drinking.

It is dangerous to allow hypomania to escalate into mania; this can result in severe exhaustion and malnutrition, or an abrupt swing into severe depression. Certainly it will mean that on recovery the patient will bitterly regret many of his actions. The events attendant upon a hypomanic episode can have a touch of comedy about them – dancing naked in front of an easily shocked neighbour; calling the doctor 'Baldy' or 'Fatty'. Sutherland (1976) recounts how he complained loudly about the shortage of canes in a sex shop. Yet the feelings of the perpetrator if he recalls these incidents later are intensely painful – the torment familiar to most of us of remembering a terrible *faux pas*, but magnified many times over. A patient who had suffered an attack of hypomania pleaded with this author, 'Please keep me locked up – don't let me do things like that again.'

We need to be alert to the aftermath of a hypomanic episode and tune in sensitively. One person may find the humour of the situation sufficient to overcome shame; another may need a great deal of reassurance that he is not held responsible and that there are no serious consequences. The *sequelae* of a spending spree sometimes require practical action by the social worker. Armed with impressive medical evidence he may be able to return some of the goods, or extricate the client from a contract. Under British law, a contract made before onset of mental disorder is binding, and so is a contract made by a person 'of unsound mind' for 'the necessaries of life' (to be defined by the court in the case of disputes). Contracts for articles other than necessaries are not binding if they would not have been made while the person was well.

Family relationships can be affected, especially if there are pre-existing problems. The social worker may be the person best placed to help, not by over-zealous problem-hunting, but by making himself available when relatives fail to visit, or hesitate to welcome the patient back, or express fear, anger or scorn. Some relatives need reassurance that they are in no way to blame for the patient's illness.

Admission to hospital is usually essential. It is surprising how many hypomanic patients can be persuaded to enter voluntarily, accepting the reality of their situation if only at one level and only for short periods at a time. The worker involved at this stage may have to struggle to find some formula whereby he and the patient can agree about the need for treatment. This might be done by suggesting that the patient needs to rest, or may like to 'get away'. There are obvious difficulties in reconciling a regard for honesty in the relationship and respect for the person, with the importance of obtaining treatment at the earliest opportunity. In interviewing the hypomanic patient the worker may find himself under considerable provocation: 'keeping one's cool', avoiding arguments, and speaking directly and firmly will help to gain the patient's co-operation.

Treatment with a major tranquilliser is fast and effective. The patient will probably be kept under observation for a while because of the need to look out for a possible depressive swing. When the patient returns home, lithium carbonate tablets are often prescribed. Lithium carbonate is a very effective means of preventing further episodes of hypomania, but the importance of regular blood checks cannot be overemphasised: if the serum lithium exceeds the therapeutic level, toxic side-effects can result (Johnson, 1974a; 1974b). As with other forms of prophylactic medication (such as phenothiazines in schizophrenia), many people object to taking drugs when they are feeling perfectly well. If a relapse occurs it is often difficult to ascertain whether the patient gave up the tablets because he was feeling 'high', or became 'high' as a result of doing so.

Many patients who have suffered from hypomania welcome the opportunity to discuss their treatment, and the sorts of changes in themselves that foreshadow a repetition of the episode. Social workers share with other staff members the responsibility to ensure that these patients are treated as responsible adults, who may well be able to monitor their own progress and seek help in advance of further trouble. With the patient's permission the relatives should also receive as much information as they feel able to assimilate. These patients and their families can be very useful treatment allies.

Hypomania is one condition for which psychological and social treatment has only a subsidiary role. Social work involvement is not often required, except when the illness causes social or personal difficulties for the patient and his family.

Depressive illness

The term 'depression' connotes normal sadness, symptoms accompanying some other mental disorder, or an illness in its own right. It is depression as an illness in its own right that we consider in this and the following chapter.

Few of us are unable to empathise with at least some of the feelings the depressed person experiences. The difference between their state of mind and 'common unhappiness', as Freud put it, seems to be one of degree rather than of kind. Yet there are pitfalls: we must beware of glib statements like 'I know how you feel', and of agreeing with the depressed person that such-and-such an event or state of affairs, or the person's past experience or behaviour, is the cause of his current distress, with the corollary that if these things can be 'worked through' all will be well again.

Talking with depressed people can be disturbing, and not only because we feel sorry for them. It seems that the things they say, and the non-verbal signals they give out, can act as stimuli that elicit painful feelings in the other person. We need to be alert to our own responses, such as trying to avoid pain by directing the conversation off certain topics because they come too close to our own concerns, or offering consolation that is more helpful for us than for the client. We should remember, too, that depressed people are usually easily tired, and that frequent brief sessions are probably more helpful than occasional long ones.

Although the psychiatrist's expertise is of central importance in the assessment of depression, the social worker needs to be able to recognise a depressive illness. Some symptoms of depression are familiar enough: sadness, low self-esteem and pessimism, frequent crying and sometimes agitated behaviour (especially in the older person). Other symptoms, however, are not part of the everyday notion of 'depression'. These include physical symptoms, such as sleep disturbance, weight loss, slowness and lack of energy some-times amounting to stupor, aches and pains, and constipation; and psychological symptoms, such as preoccupation with health, poor memory, indecisiveness, irritability and obsessions (repetitive un-wanted thoughts). The person may experience feelings of depersona-lisation (not feeling real), or derealisation (the world takes on a dreamlike quality). Delusions of guilt, illness or poverty, and audi-tory hallucinations may also occur.

It is hard to know where to draw the dividing line between the depression that requires urgent psychiatric referral and possibly hospital care, and the depression that does not. No clear guidelines can be offered, except the cliché, 'if in doubt seek the advice of a more experienced professional'. However, the next section, which deals with the classification of depression, may help – not only towards a better understanding of the terminology and decision-making processes of psychiatrists, but also towards greater confidence on the social worker's part when he is involved in helping a person who shows symptoms of depression.

The classification of depression

There is much controversy concerning the classification of depression. Some authorities believe it to be one disorder ranging along a continuum (or along several continua), while others claim there are two separate disorders with distinctively different causes, symptoms and suitable approaches to treatment. This is not the place to elaborate on the arguments for and against each point of view. However, it is important for the social worker to understand the distinctions, based on types of symptom and beliefs about causation, because these usually affect the choice of treatment and the contributions of the different helping professions. What follows is a brief account of three dimensions along which people suffering from depression may be assessed. The three dimensions are different systems for categorising the symptoms of depression, and may therefore be seen as three separate approaches to diagnosis.

(1) *Endogenous–reactive (or exogenous)*. 'Endogenous' means 'arising from within', and refers to depression apparently 'coming out of the blue'. 'Reactive' means brought about by events, usually loss or stress.

The distinction rests primarily on a judgement about causation: if no obvious precipitating factor can be found, or if the patient's misery is considered to be totally out of proportion to his situation, then endogenous depression may be diagnosed. This will be even more likely if his symptoms include a high proportion of physical symptoms, such as stupor, weight loss, or constipation. If, on the other hand, the presence of recent loss or intolerable life circumstances is noted, then the 'reactive' designation is more probable, especially if the symptoms are predominantly mental rather than physical.

(2) *Psychotic–neurotic*. This distinction closely resembles the previous one. However, the emphasis is rather on whether or not contact with reality is preserved, and on distance from 'normality'.

Willis (1976) lists the features differentiating neurosis from psychosis as follows: (a) preservation of contact with reality, that is, no symptoms such as hallucinations, delusions, thought-disorder or intellectual impairment; (b) symptoms of anxiety common, whether somatic or psychological; (c) minor mood disturbance; (d) symptoms tend to be mild and chronic; (e) insight, that is, awareness of illness is common, though the implications of illness in terms of unconscious conflict, etc. are not readily available to insight; (f) personality change does not occur.

Priest (Priest and Steinert, 1977) gives a useful summary of the key differences between neurotic and psychotic depression: the person with neurotic depression does not suffer such severe retardation; he may be preoccupied with disease, guilt and so on, but he wonders rather than believes that he is seriously ill or grievously at fault.

(3) *Severe–mild*. Although this distinction is less often discussed in the textbooks, it probably provides the most useful framework for consideration of the psychiatrist's choice of treatment, the social worker's role, and other key questions, such as whether hospital admission is needed. Simply put, the severely depressed person is unable to look after himself, his general health is suffering, and there may be a risk that he will injure himself (or very rarely, someone else as well). He may have symptoms of the psychotic type, he may be so retarded as to appear totally stuporous, or else he may be very agitated. He may express extreme mental distress, perhaps hinting that he is considering suicide.

Some depressive illnesses begin mild, and become severe; others remain mild throughout their course. A severe depression may become mild, or else change abruptly into hypomania.

From this short account it can be seen that the three diagnostic continua are three different ways of describing a given depression. The terms 'endogenous', 'psychotic', and 'severe' are often, but not always, interchangeable. An endogenous depression need not be severe, though a psychotic one always is. A reactive or neurotic depression can be severe.

Assessment and the start of intervention in severe depression

In view of the wide range of symptoms, possible causative factors, and the variety of potential treatment approaches, assessment needs to be a multi-disciplinary endeavour. The first task is to assess the person's illness in terms of the different typologies outlined above. To this end the social worker will contribute his own observations of the person, his everyday behaviour, and the family's account of the changes they have observed. Special attention needs to be paid to any indications of the possibility of suicide (see pp. 56–8). The social history will cover personal relationships, past and current experiences of loss and stress, some estimate of what the person has to cope with, and how well he has coped in the past.

Psychiatrists differ considerably in how much interest they take in the search for causes. Aetiology is as much in dispute as is classification; and heredity, biochemistry, childhood experience and present circumstances have each been considered paramount by different authors, either in one particular type of depression or in depression in general. However, most psychiatrists will pay particular attention to a family history of depression – especially if the illness is episodic, or alternating with hypomania (suggesting the endogenous type) – and also to accounts of recent loss or severe life difficulties (suggesting the reactive type).

In general, the more the illness fits an endogenous or psychotic picture – and particularly if the patient has suffered from hypomania – the more likely it is that a genetic or physical-causation theory will be favoured; and further, the more likely it is that the psychiatrist will opt for a physical-treatment approach. But some psychiatrists regularly suggest physical treatment first, whatever the classification or suspected cause. Perhaps the only generalisation that can be made with any confidence is that depression alternating with hypomania, and depression that closely fits the endogenous or the psychotic type, will almost invariably be treated by physical methods; when depression is judged to be severe this will also be the case, although if it appears to be reactive or neurotic in quality, physical treatment is less usual, and other kinds of help are commonly given. The rest of this chapter describes the physical treatments for depression, and the next chapter deals with psychological and social approaches.

Physical treatment of depression

There is strong evidence for the efficacy of drug treatment in depression. Three major drug groups are currently in use: the mono-amine oxidase inhibitors (MAOIs), the tricyclics, and lithium carbonate (the latter prescribed as a prophylactic, as for the patient with recurrent hypomania). The MAOIs can interact with certain other drugs and foodstuffs to produce a dangerous rise in blood pressure, and the patient is always given a list of banned substances along with his prescription. Other key points for the non-medical helper to remember are that all these drugs take some time to work – a matter of two to three weeks; that all of them can have unpleasant side-effects; and that several drugs may have to be tried before the psychiatrist is satisfied that the best remedy has been found for the individual. After the patient has recovered, the prescription is usually continued for some months in order to prevent relapse.

When drug treatment is ineffective, or is considered to be too slow (for example, when a serious suicide risk is suspected), electro-convulsive therapy (ECT) may be given instead. The usual procedure is for the patient to receive a muscle relaxant and a general anaesthetic; then two electrodes are fastened to the temples and a small electric current is administered. The patient is usually awake within fifteen minutes. He may suffer temporary memory loss and confusion, and some patients also have a headache but there is no firm evidence of long-lasting harm, and the danger is the same as for other forms of medical intervention carried out under a general anaesthetic.

Most psychiatrists (and many patients) believe ECT to be the most effective treatment for the type of depression called endogenous (characterised by somatic symptoms and lack of obvious precipitating factors); and no one who has worked in a psychiatric unit can deny that many patients who are mute and severely retarded can be returned to a normal state after two or three ECT treatments over just a few days. ECT in some cases can literally save lives: prior to its introduction, death from malnutrition was not uncommon among severely depressed patients. The rigorous research review by the American Psychiatric Association (1978) concluded that ECT is a 'very effective anti-depressant treatment' and that 'certain depressed patients will respond to ECT and not to anti-depressant drugs'. Recently, a social scientist (Garfield, 1979), and a psychiatrist (Crow, 1979), have both reached a similar conclusion, although noting that abuses exist, both in the manner it is given and the selection of patients who receive it. In what was probably the best controlled trial yet conducted (Johnstone *et al.*, 1980), the conclusions were somewhat less clear cut. The comparison was between real and simulated ECT (both groups receiving intensive nursing care). ECT was significantly more effective in the very short term, but the patients who did not receive it showed an equal degree of improvement two months after the beginning of the four weeks' treatment. Memory tests showed that impairment caused by ECT was short-lived.

Most psychiatrists use ECT sparingly and with care, reserving it for patients who are profoundly disturbed or retarded, those who do not respond to drugs, and those whose circumstances make a rapid recovery particularly important. But its use is a matter of concern to many social workers.

When there is reason to believe that someone is being given ECT against his will and illegally, the social worker might consider seeking advice from a patients' rights organisation. But in most situations expressing one's doubts about this treatment to the patient (who will usually follow his doctor's advice in any case) will probably do more harm than good.

Many patients recover completely after drugs or ECT, and in these cases, as with hypomania, social work involvement may be minimal. Those social workers who are involved with the severely depressed person and his family can best help by giving support and encouragement, perhaps helping to clear up misunderstandings between family members (the patient may have been very hard to live with). Sometimes clients who are depressed will propose making drastic changes in their life, such as separation from their spouse or resignation from work. In these circumstances, the social worker should do all he can to dissuade them from taking major decisions at a time when their judgement is probably affected by depression.

The social worker's role is very different in those cases where the depressed person does not respond to physical treatment, or relapses frequently despite prophylactic medication; or where bereavement or some other form of loss, a difficult social situation, or a longstanding personality problem are clearly implicated. The psycho-social models of depression can be helpful in construing these cases, and the intervention procedures that follow from them may involve the social worker in a central role.Where such a model fits, social or psychological intervention along the lines discussed in the next chapter ought to be considered. However, many authorities would recommend conservatism in planning the intervention, reserving the broad-spectrum approach for those patients who do not respond to medical treatment and whose depression is very obviously related to personal troubles. In any case, the severely depressed person is unlikely to be able to take his part in the work required in a psychological approach until the intensity of his symptoms has been mitigated.

4

Psychological and Social Approaches to Depression

All the psycho-social treatments appear to offer comfort, the possibility of a lasting improvement in functioning, and respect for the person as an individual, and to be harmless in comparison with the somatic treatments described in the previous chapter. But after thorough examination of their merits and demerits, Priest (Priest and Steinert, 1977) suggests that in *severe* depression even the least intensive – offering empathy and encouraging the person to talk – can be too much for the patient to cope with; to go further and attempt to 'change personality' by offering 'insight' might do harm. An active behavioural or cognitive approach may be equally inappropriate. Unjustified faith in these methods can lead to neglect of effective and urgently required medical intervention, so that the person's physical health deteriorates through self-neglect, or his despair deepens to the point of suicide. Two cases known to this author highlight this last point. After his wife had left him, a social work client became very tearful, stopped going to work, and talked of doing away with himself. The social worker refused to apply for compulsory hospital admission; she was on call over the weekend, and was confident that the man would feel able to contact her if he felt desperate. The man made no attempt to seek anyone's help, and cut his throat. Another man, who suffered depressive episodes about once every two years, and had previously responded rapidly to ECT, noted the onset of his symptoms and asked to be treated again as before. Instead, he was admitted to a therapeutic community ward, and pressed to examine his past and current problems in a group discussion. At the end of the first meeting he left the hospital and took a fatal overdose.

In addition to such hazards, we should remember that the depressed patient who begins a course of physical treatment with apparently every reason for wanting to die, every possible personality and social problem, may well turn out to be perfectly able to run his life and to experience satisfaction in his work and social roles. In the depths of depression people feel unloved and undeserving, and are often preoccupied with the very topics that are central to the content of 'talking treatment'; their behaviour as well as their talk may be affected, so that they appear to lack important life skills, especially social skills. This picture can be very misleading, and sometimes intrusive and unnecessary 'helping' can ensue.

However, a psycho-social treatment approach may be appropriate alongside drug therapy or ECT, or may follow a course of medical treatment. If the depression is not severe, and is very obviously related to circumstances or to longstanding personality or relationship problems, psycho-social treatment alone will be the logical intervention choice.

Taking first that hard-to-define social work activity 'support', and bearing in mind Priest's warning that not every depressed patient can benefit even from this, we should note that some authorities have suggested that support is best directed towards encouraging compliance with a drug regime! Beyond this, it seems reasonable to assume that those patients who are chronically though mildly depressed may gain comfort from the chance to talk with a sympathetic person, and may need practical help and encouragement in order to cope with their 'problems of living'. There is some evidence in favour of 'supportive casework' with depressed patients in improving their social functioning (Weissman *et al.*, 1974), but the improvement did not extend to their depressive symptoms, and casework did not prevent relapse. In a later study, this research group found casework (described as 'psychotherapy') to be as effective as drugs (Weissman *et al.*, 1979). However, both studies have been criticised by Clare (1980) with regard to the assessment methods used.

It may be appropriate to offer a more focused type of help. In this chapter we consider depression from several points of view: as a reaction to inner conflict or to loss; as a cluster of learned behaviours and a learned mental set; as a response to a combination of socially determined disadvantages; and as a reaction to processes within the family system. The divisions are somewhat artificial, since these viewpoints can complement one another, and in many cases the interventions derived from them turn out to be quite similar in practice, despite their being associated with different schools of theory and therapy. This said, the social worker may find it helpful to consider each approach separately and to assess whether it seems to fit the individual case.

Psychodynamic approaches

According to one psychoanalytical view, depression is a condition in which unacceptable feelings of guilt or anger are not overtly expressed, but are turned inwards. These feelings are associated with an early loss experience. The person feels that his destructive urges have driven away someone he loved but was also ambivalent towards, or else he feels angry with the lost person for deserting him. More recent losses reawaken these feelings. The fact that depression is more common among those who were bereaved or separated from a parent during childhood is cited in support of this view, as well as the psychoanalytical investigations of individual patients, beginning with those of Freud.

Following from this, the treatment that is advocated is psychoanalysis or psychodynamic psychotherapy. These approaches seek to provide the person with an opportunity to develop understanding, and hence conscious mastery, of the causes of his current difficulties, by 'working through' his past experiences, which are exerting a distorted or exaggerated influence upon his functioning.' (For detailed discussion of the theories and practice of psychoanalytic psychotherapy see, for example, Mendelsohn, 1974; Arieti and Bemporad, 1980.)

It is generally accepted that the style of casework that comes close to psychotherapy as practised by a qualified psychotherapist requires special training. Social workers who lack this training can take comfort from such findings as those of Strupp and Hadley (1979) which, although derived from research on 'neurotic' students, might be generalisable to depressed adults as well. In this study, it was found that psychoanalytical or experiential therapy was no more effective than talks with an untrained 'therapist', and that focus on the present, and advice and encouragement to take part in activities, were associated with a good outcome, whereas long silences, and talking about the past, were not.

On the whole, the verdict as to the effectiveness of psychodynamic psychotherapy must remain 'not proven', although it is difficult to balance conflicting claims (or indeed to find an unbiased reviewer of this literature).

Clare's (1980) conclusion that psychotherapy seems to add little to the effects of drug treatment would appear to sum up the view of those authorities who take empirical research as the best test of effectiveness.

Nevertheless, some social workers will feel that for some of their depressed clients only professional psychoanalytical psychotherapy will serve, and some will want to press for this on the client's behalf. Bloch's (1979) list of patient-characteristics favourable for long-term insight-oriented psychotherapy includes the presence of depression. His other criteria are as follows: (a) a reasonable level of personality integration; (b) motivation for change; (c) realistic expectations of the therapeutic processes involved, reflecting 'psychological mindedness'; (d) at least average intelligence; (e) non-psychotic condition; (f) life circumstances free of any unresolvable crises. Schofield (1964) summarised the 'good prognosis' variables as YAVIS: Young, Attractive, Verbal, Intelligent, Successful; and a negative version is given by Goldstein and Simonson (1971): Homely, Old, Unattractive, Non-verbal, Dumb (HOUND). Unfortunately, the same factors operate in respect of most psychological treatment approaches!

Depression as grief

This approach has much in common with the psychodynamic approach, and it too was originally formulated by psychoanalysts. The question, 'Is grief a disease?', was answered in the affirmative by Engel (1961); certainly there is no clear-cut dividing line between the psychological and somatic 'symptoms' of the recently bereaved person and those of the depressed patient.

For normal grief, the person requires only the support necessary to carry out his current tasks. His general practitioner may prescribe a small amount of tranquillisers if he is too upset to cope, but otherwise professional help is not needed. For people without the support of relatives or close friends, bereavement counselling is carried out by volunteers in some areas, with the aim of providing understanding and reassurance as the person goes through the normal phases of mourning. The phases are: shock, disbelief or denial, anger, guilt and despair, followed by resolution, which is defined as a realistic acceptance of the loss and a return to normal functioning – taking up new roles, perhaps, and making new relationships. There is some evidence that this kind of help can prevent later depression (Raphael, 1977).

Professional help becomes appropriate when someone gets stuck at a particular stage, or fails to reach the resolution stage; and this is more likely if the loss was unexpected, if it has far-reaching consequences, or if the relationship with the dead person was ambivalent. One problem with this model is that the stages do not necessarily occur in the order in which they are usually placed. (For this reason, recent theorists such as Ramsay and Happee (1977) prefer to speak of 'components' rather than 'stages'.) This adds to the difficulty in recognising when a grief reaction should be considered pathological and the person in need of professional help. A waiting period of one year has been proposed as a guide. Examples of pathological failure to reach resolution include the person who remains deeply distressed after this period has elapsed, the woman who insists years later that a husband who has abandoned her will return, and the mother who devotes herself to thinking and talking about her dead child while neglecting her other children. Sometimes the person does not himself bring the loss to our attention: what looks like a depressive illness coming 'out of the blue' may constitute an anniversary reaction, or may be triggered by association in an apparently unconnected set of circumstances.

Helping these clients means giving them the opportunity to talk freely and to experience the normal components of mourning in an atmosphere of acceptance. By giving permission, and by guiding the person through the various stages, the worker gradually helps him to reach the conclusion of the process. Then the focus turns outwards again, away from the loss and the past and the mourner's painful feelings, and on to his current networks and tasks, and future plans. In finding new roles, and working towards new goals, a task-centred or a behavioural approach may be helpful. Lindemann's (1944) discussion remains a useful set of guidelines to the first or 'grieving' part of the work, and for the later part we can draw on the general literature of social casework.

A behavioural variant of assisted grief work has been proposed by Ramsay (1976). His method seems especially suitable for the person who is denying the loss, or who remains incapacitated by distress long after it occurred. The therapist obliges the patient to face up to his loss intensively over a matter of a few days, experiencing the most painful reminders over and over again, and saying 'I will never see her again', and 'She is in a grave', and so on, until the powerful emotions have been first evoked and then extinguished. This procedure is extremely painful for both the therapist and the client, and Ramsay warns against allowing therapy to cease before the process is complete. It seems that clients agreeing to this treatment have to be exceptionally motivated, and that great care must be taken to guard against the risk of suicide. It is of interest in this context because of its similarity to the style of helping suggested by Lindemann and other psychodynamically oriented writers. Ramsay provides evidence of its value for those individuals whom he has treated, as well as a convincing rationale.

There are certain difficulties with the model of depression as grief. As we have seen, it does not provide precise guidelines as to when a grief reaction should be considered 'pathological'. It also begs certain questions about people's 'adjustment' to loss: some losses, surely, cannot be forgotten or compensated for. If, for example, during a history-taking interview, the client is strongly reminded of great unhappiness in the past, and then has difficulty talking about it or becomes upset, should we therefore assume that the subject needs to be reopened and gone over again? Olshansky (1962) maintains that chronic sorrow is the normal state of parents who have a mentally-handicapped child; if this is so, can one logically expect to guide them through to a resolution stage? Finally, we should beware of assuming that every loss suffered by a person who later develops depression is necessarily 'unresolved'. Losses are 'life events', and these play a role in precipitating depressive illness as well as other forms of illness (Brown *et al.*, 1973; Paykel *et al.*, 1969). Although much has been written on this theme, we should perhaps be conservative in construing all types of depression as merely reaction to loss, even when major losses have occurred in the depressed person's life.

Learning and cognitive theories

The models and intervention strategies developed by learning and cognitive theorists are numerous, and depression is a major focus for their research at the present time. In this section, three approaches are discussed. They are compatible with one another, and the styles of treatment they suggest are often very similar.

Several learning theorists have construed depression as the result of lack or loss of positive reinforcement (for example, Lewinsohn, 1974). It may have developed after the loss of a major source of reinforcement or of cues for behaviour leading to reinforcement, as when a husband or wife dies or leaves; or it may be due to lack of skills to obtain reinforcement, as in the case of a person who does not have the ability to make new friends. The key to helping is to find ways for the person to obtain positive reinforcement once again. In some cases the worker will be involved in 'getting things' for the client; more often it will mean helping the person to get things for himself. According to this simple but sensible model, the first step is a careful analysis of what is lacking and what avenues are open to the person. Sometimes straightforward advice is all that is needed: an introduction to a social club, a list of evening classes, or welfare-rights information, may set the person in the right direction. A more complex intervention is usually necessary, however.

In the search for tasks likely to bring success, the client's desires and skills have to be taken into account. Not everyone wants a hectic social life or more leisure interests; and a person who lacks social skills will not find a girlfriend no matter how many eligible young women he meets.

Many depressed patients do lack social skills (Trower *et al.*, 1978), and have fewer friends than those who are not depressed (Henderson, 1977). But it is often hard to decide whether this problem is partly a cause of depression or whether it is a consequence. After other treatments have been given, and the person remains depressed, is still unable to hold a conversation, is not rewarding company, and cannot ask other people for things he wants, then a social skills training approach is worth trying (see Chapter 5). The results of evaluative studies of this approach with various groups of psychiatric patients, including some diagnosed as depressed, have been encouraging (Marzillier, 1978; Argyle *et al.*, 1974).

Besides a deficit in social skills, the client may lack other abilities, to the extent that he is unable to reach his goals, and other kinds of skill deficits will require other kinds of help. Marital therapy may be needed if the central problem lies in the person's relationship with husband or wife, family therapy if in parent–child communication.

Learning to cope with the family finances, to organise a journey, to read and write, are all possible way-stages between the position of being without and that of obtaining one's goals. Anxiety, as distinct from a basic lack of skills, may be the chief obstacle, and in that case the worker will first aim to remove the anxiety (see Chapter 5).

To sum up: the somewhat simplistic operant model of depression leads to the application of a wide variety of different helping strategies, according to a detailed analysis of the client's goals and abilities.

Before turning to more sophisticated psychological models, we should note in passing that some behavioural practitioners have worked directly with so-called 'depressive behaviours'. It often seems as though they are dealing with 'moaning', rather than 'depression'. The client who is constantly complaining is given a thorough change of environmental contingencies: family and friends stop rewarding the complaints, and only attend to constructive talk and action, so that the 'depressive behaviour' is gradually given up (Liberman and Raskin, 1971).

Another behavioural approach is to focus on emotional aspects of depression, construing them as reactions to painful stimuli, and treating them in a similar manner to anxiety reactions (McAuley and Quinn, 1971). Thus, the person who becomes distressed upon visiting a happily married couple because he is reminded of a broken relationship, or the woman who has lost her baby and is upset at the sight of other women's babies, might be helped by gradual exposure to these situations.

A more complex and more 'cognitive' theory is Seligman's 'learned helplessness' (Seligman, 1975). This theory states that the feelings and behaviour that make up depression result from a cognitive set involving the belief that one can do nothing to change the environment – in other words, the individual's responses will not lead to reinforcement; and this comes about as a consequence of experiencing uncontrollable trauma. This may be a recent experience; but a history of lack of control may predispose the person to becoming helpless. The person who has become helpless requires the experience of being effectual again in order to alter his belief that there is nothing he can do to change his world. Such experience has to be gradual and positive, lest new failures should arise to intensify his feeling of helplessness. Seligman once told this author (who was making rather ambitious plans for a group of depressed housewives in a deprived area), 'Don't ask your depressed clients to tackle the Town Hall – just help them into their coats and encourage them to go to the local bingo club.'

A treatment programme based on Seligman's model could look identical to the kinds of programme already discussed. The main difference is that the emphasis must *always* be on the client's own efforts, ensuring that these bring rewards, and on a step-by-step approach with a great deal of encouragement.

Other workers in the cognitive-behavioural group, of whom the best known is Beck (1974), focus particularly on the thinking of the depressed person, postulating that depressive thoughts precede depressive feelings and behaviour. They therefore set out to train the person to alter his own thought patterns – first to pinpoint and monitor them, then to substitute more rational and constructive self-statements, and to give himself some form of reinforcement (a sort of mental pat on the back) for doing this. The three main areas addressed (known as Beck's Cognitive Triad) are negative views of oneself, of the world, and of the future. The client is also encouraged to test out his beliefs, to see if his gloomy predictions are confirmed in reality. This form of treatment is being developed and evaluated in several centres, but training is still difficult to obtain. If the promising results so far reported (for example, Rush *et al.*, 1977) continue to be confirmed, we are likely to see a growth in cognitive-therapy training opportunities. Experience so far suggests that this method is appropriate for those depressed clients who are not severely ill, who suffer a chronic depressive condition, and who do not also show an admixture of anxiety. This generalisation is probably true for the other behavioural approaches to depression as well, although these have as yet received little research scrutiny, despite well-documented reports of single cases.

In concluding this section, it is worth noting that, because of their compatibility with one another, and the fact that each of these models seems suited to some clients, workers such as Lewinsohn now combine them in one cognitive-behavioural model of depression, and select techniques for whichever aspect of depression seems to be most prominent in the individual case. Thus the to-and-fro interaction among thoughts, feelings, and behavioural excesses and deficits, is recognised, and intervention begins at the level that the worker and the client choose as the most promising starting point.

The social-origins approach

A group of sociologists, following a large-scale and meticulous study of women, have advanced a model of depression that is in no way contradictory to the psychological models outlined above (Brown and Harris, 1978). They link depression (both depression of a degree calling for medical treatment, and a sub-clinical level as well) to certain key variables, some of which are described as 'provoking agents' and others as 'vulnerability factors'. The 'provoking agents' are severe 'life events' of the kind identified in previous research by Brown and other workers (Brown *et al.*, 1973; Paykel *et al.*, 1969), such as bereavement, or losing one's home, and major ongoing difficulties such as housing or financial problems. However, it is usually only in combination with vulnerability factors that these events and difficulties bring about depressive illness. The vulnerability factors are: loss of mother before the age of eleven; three or more children in the family under fourteen; lack of a confiding relationship; and lack of paid employment. The difference between working-class and middle-class women (four times as many of the former develop a depressive illness if they experience a provoking agent) is due to the greater likelihood of the working-class woman experiencing the vulnerability factors. Brown and Harris consider that the vulnerability factors are basic causes of a sense of low self-esteem, which paves the way for depression in the face of adverse life circumstances.

The intervention proposed by these workers is preventive, and at a societal level: more opportunities for women to go out to work, adequate child-care facilities such as day-nurseries, and better financial and housing provision. They do not accept that there is an endogenous type of depression, and suggest that if their proposals for social change were carried out, the rate of depressive illness among women would decrease considerably.

The conclusions of Brown and his colleagues fit in with Seligman's view, that poverty and poor housing and other forms of deprivation predispose people to helplessness; with Beck's account of depressive thinking; and with Lewinsohn's view of the depressed person as someone who lacks reinforcement. Nevertheless, this research requires replication with other populations before its somewhat sweeping conclusions can be accepted as the final word on depression. Meanwhile, it is certainly a model that fits many of the depressed and deprived young mothers who become social work clients. It highlights the need for social work to join with other helping professions to seek social change at a local and national level. It also suggests guidelines for intervention in individual cases: encouragement and help to find work, perhaps part-time, and arranging for substitute care for children. Marital therapy might be helpful in an attempt to improve communication between wives and husbands, and facilitating social activities might enable women to find a substitute 'confiding relationship' outside of marriage. Is it going beyond the evidence to an unacceptable extent to suggest that regular support from a social worker might also serve this purpose?

Depression and the family

There has been little well-designed research on family interaction and its relation to depression, apart from the findings concerning the importance of a close confiding relationship (Brown and Harris, 1978). The other models discussed above might illuminate the assessment of the depressed person's family environment in a variety of respects: drawing our attention to families who provide little reinforcement or do little to encourage positive action (the operant model); relatives who seem to encourage the kinds of negative thinking described by Beck, or who 'take control' and prevent the helpless person from regaining a sense of efficacy. Vaughn and Leff (1976) have obtained some evidence to suggest that the 'high expressed emotion' home is as harmful for the depressed patient as it is for the schizophrenic patient: indeed, high levels of criticism may hurt the depressed person more than the schizophrenic, perhaps because he is less able to withdraw to shield himself, and also because criticism from others finds echoes in his own view of himself.

Ways of helping might include the same approaches as were outlined in the chapter on schizophrenia, but they should be applied with caution. Like the families of schizophrenic patients these families suffer a considerable burden, and to propose family therapy might be unnecessarily intrusive. Only if there is very good reason to suppose that family interaction plays a central role should we consider intervention to change the behaviour of family members. Offers of family or marital therapy can sound like accusations to both the family and the patient, and might increase despair and guilt in the depressed person; some carefully designed research suggests that social casework directed at marital problems, though it may be helpful with the marital problems, may not reduce the depressive symptoms (Friedman, 1975; Gibbons *et al.*, 1978).

Throughout this chapter, it has been emphasised that much research has yet to be done, before we can be truly confident that social and psychological treatments for depression are effective by comparison with the effects of time or medical treatment. However, there is every reason to pursue some of the goals that have been mentioned for their own sake: the provision of better opportunities for women to choose to work if they wish to, and better living conditions for the poor; the reduction of family discord; and the learning of new skills, which will widen the choices people have in their lives and help them to develop an increased sense of mastery. And the effectiveness debate is far from settled yet.

McAuley (1980), reviewing the literature on psychological treatments for depression, comments that although there is as yet no evidence that they are more effective than drugs,

> care must be taken prior to reaching premature conclusions. The long-term as well as the short-term effects must be considered. It is possible that some forms of psychotherapeutic techniques, while they may not help in the short term, may go some way to stimulating an improved long-term prognosis.

A rapid reduction in depressive symptoms is not the only important goal.

5

Anxiety States and Phobias

Anxiety states and phobias are very common forms of neurosis.

'Neurosis' is a broad category of psychiatric disorders, ranging from the severely disabling to the mild and transient. The majority of people suffering from neurosis are general-practice patients rather than psychiatrists' patients, and there is no clear dividing line between the neurotic and the normal.

Aetiology is much disputed, but most authorities would agree that neurotic symptoms arise as a result of maladaptive learning or as a reaction to stress. The stress may be external: for example, the threat of being deserted by one's spouse; or internal (perhaps unconscious): for example, an unresolved loss or a conflict between inner drives. 'Anxiety' is generally seen as a central feature of neurosis. Authors of the psychoanalytic school write of 'anxiety' as an unconscious motivator – the surface symptoms representing a compromise solution to a conflict between different forces within the personality, which solution serves to protect the person from experiencing anxiety. But as Willis (1976) comments, 'it is absurd to talk of "unconscious anxiety" since anxiety is by definition a subjective experience and terms such as "unconscious anxiety" are catchall phrases used to conceal ignorance'. Much the same could be said of related concepts, such as 'unconscious conflict'.

Genetic, personality and constitutional factors are also implicated, perhaps in giving certain people a propensity to develop symptoms in the face of difficulties (for a brief review, see Marks, 1973). It seems as though each of us is vulnerable to becoming 'neurotic' under stress; our vulnerability varies not only according to our long-term attributes, but also according to the state of our physical health. There is also some interesting research that suggests that chronic neurosis in one partner in a marriage can 'infect' the other partner over the course of time (Kreitman *et al.*, 1970; 1971; Ovenstone, 1973).

In Chapter 3 I mentioned the several ways in which depression is classified – psychotic or neurotic, endogenous or reactive, severe or mild – and the controversy as to whether it is one illness or two separate illnesses. The severe–mild continuum was chosen as a convenient framework for discussion, and the description of models and approaches in Chapter 4 concerned mainly the milder conditions and those which have passed from a severe into a mild stage. 'Mild', 'reactive', and 'psychological' depressions are often classified as neurotic disorders, that is, those which show fewer physical symptoms, do not involve delusions or lack of insight, and do not respond so well to physical treatments.

'Depressive neurosis' is often found in association with another set of neurotic symptoms, especially anxiety states and agoraphobia, but also in several of the less common syndromes described in Chapter 6. The diagnosis is then sometimes given as 'mixed neurosis', but this is avoided as far as possible because most psychiatrists will want to prescribe specific treatments for the separate conditions. However, the 'mixed neurosis' is sufficiently common for there to be numerous research reports concerning patients classified in this way, and there are combined antidepressant-anxiolytic drugs.

Anxiety

Anxiety too may be part of a 'mixed neurosis' with another type of neurotic disorder. As a disorder in its own right it takes two main forms – anxiety states, and phobias (the latter also called 'situational anxiety'). The term 'anxiety', of course, refers to several different symptoms; and it may accompany any other mental disorder, as an extra complication of schizophrenia and organic disorders, among others. This is hardly surprising since anxiety is a universal reaction to threatening situations.

Thus, anxiety like depression is something that we can all empathise with – or we think we can. It is usually the circumstances in which it occurs, rather than the feeling itself, that we judge to be abnormal. However, anxiety at its most severe is something that few of us have experienced. Leonard (1927) described it as 'the acutest agony of the conscious brain', and Sutherland (1976) writes: 'I would not have believed it possible to feel such extreme anxiety. My heart pounded, my body shook, my stomach felt as though all the blood had drained away, and my legs felt too weak to carry me.' Leonard is describing a short-lived panic attack in the context of a phobic disorder, but Sutherland spent days in this condition before a powerful tranquillising drug was prescribed for him.

Anxiety symptoms are psychological (the person's appraisal of his situation, a feeling of fear, sometimes amounting to an overwhelming sense of dread), physiological (faintness, sweating, rapid pulse, shaking, difficulty in breathing, muscle tension, nausea, digestive upsets) and behavioural (running away, avoidance). They are all part of normal experience at some time or other: the near-miss when driving, entering the examination room, the arrival of a telegram; but for the patient with an anxiety state or a phobia they cause continuing misery, and interfere with work and social relationships, and basic everyday activities, such as eating and sleeping. These varying types of symptoms do not always occur together, nor does relief from one necessarily mean relief from the others. This is why it is necessary to consider all of them in assessment, treatment, and monitoring the person's recovery. Also, as Lader (1978) demonstrates in his model of anxiety, the physiological ones feed into the psychological, and so on, back and forth.

To a greater or lesser degree the person with an anxiety state suffers the full range of symptoms, except the escape and avoidance behaviour. Panic attacks may occur from time to time but the person is chronically in the state Sutherland describes.

In agoraphobia there are often panic attacks, followed by avoidance involving more and more different situations as time goes on, and often the chronic features of the anxiety state as well. In the other phobias the person avoids a specific feared object or situation, and may not suffer the other symptoms except when he meets with the phobic stimulus.

As well as suffering from the anxiety symptoms themselves, the person carries the additional burden of knowing that his reaction is either irrational ('there is nothing to be anxious about'), or disproportionate ('I ought to be able to cope with this'). He often fails to attract sympathy from other people unless he complains of physiological symptoms. Many patients try to conceal their anxiety from outsiders, sometimes even from close friends or relatives. Social workers often come across agoraphobic housewives who have been house-bound for many years, and people crippled with anxiety who can only cope with their work by heroic exercise of self-control and at the expense of most other facets of their lives.

Anxiety states, and to an even greater extent, agoraphobia, can have serious effects on the life of the whole family. Husbands are called home from work when their wives have a panic attack, children may be burdened with errands and escort duties, or even prevented from attending school. Social life may be restricted, with resulting dissatisfaction and isolation. The families of agoraphobics are sometimes said to be over-solicitous, and have been suspected of obtaining some benefit for themselves out of the patient's difficulties. It is true that they are often tolerant, perhaps too tolerant, but the rest does not necessarily follow and there is little evidence for supposing that this is a general pattern. Nor should we assume without evidence that there are marital problems which are being coped with or reflected by the patient's symptoms: in our present state of knowledge it is not possible to make generalisations about the relationship between marital interaction and the development of neurosis (Marks, 1973). This is a very individualised matter, but it is probably fair to say that the hypothesis that there are concealed family or marital problems is not a good starting point for intervention.

Treatment

Anxiolytic drugs are commonly prescribed, especially benzodiazepines. Indeed this drug group, the minor tranquillisers, are the most frequently prescribed of all types of medication. In high doses, these drugs have minor side-effects, such as drowsiness and dizziness. In the long term, there is some risk of dependency. Even more serious, some clinicians fear that in some cases (as yet there seems to be no way of predicting which ones), the benzodiazepines may precipitate disinhibition and aggressive outbursts. If this proves to be correct, anyone who is working with, say, a mother of young children has cause for serious concern.

As is the case of neurotic depression, anxiety states and phobias are treated by a variety of psychological methods, many of which can involve a social worker in an ancillary or a direct-treatment role. Since the preferred approach differs according to the particular condition, we shall take specific phobias, social phobias, agoraphobia, and anxiety states separately.

Specific phobias are the easiest to treat of the four conditions, and although something as apparently trivial as a spider phobia can in fact be severely handicapping, it is very rare for the sufferer to enter hospital. The psychoanalytic approach has been abandoned by most psychiatrists in favour of a simpler, fast-acting behavioural treatment. There are two main methods – 'desensitisation' and 'flooding' – and both have impressive research backing (Marks, 1978). In desensitisation (also known as slow exposure) the client experiences the anxiety-provoking stimulus in doses of increasing intensity while feeling relaxed. This may be accomplished by first teaching him deep muscle relaxation, then taking him step-by-step through a hierarchy of items or scenes from the least to the most distressing, and finally getting him to confront the feared object or situation in real life. The method that includes all these components is called 'systematic desensitisation'. It is now known that the key factor in the process is the real-life exposure, and that the means of achieving this is not important. Many people can start right away with real-life practice, and the presence of a trusted companion may be a satisfactory substitute for relaxation. Occasionally, a tranquillising drug is used to facilitate the process. The effectiveness of desensitisation is enhanced by modelling (demonstration) – not of absolutely fearless behaviour, but of 'coping', that is, recognising that one is not totally unafraid but rather admitting that there is a difficulty to be overcome. Modelling with a 'coping' commentary merges with the cognitive-behaviour therapy procedure of teaching the client a more constructive way of talking to himself as he tackles problems. It is also important to arrange incentives and rewards for trying, and the patient's family may be asked to help with this, especially if they have been inclined to reinforce sick-role behaviour with affection and concern, while paying little attention to attempts to get better.

Social workers with behavioural training, particularly if they already have a good relationship with the client and the family, are in a favourable position to offer this kind of help.

An alternative behavioural approach is 'flooding' (rapid exposure). It is quicker, at least as effective as desensitisation for specific phobias, and more effective than desensitisation for agoraphobia;

but it may be too demanding for some patients to accept. In flooding, the patient faces the anxiety-provoking situation all at once, either first in imagination and then in reality, or in reality right away. This procedure can be made more tolerable with the use of drugs, and requires prior medical screening; it is probably not appropriate for social workers to carry out. (Stern (1978) gives a clear and detailed account of both flooding and desensitisation, and the latter point is inferred from his recommendations.) When flooding is the chosen treatment, the social worker can still play a useful role in working with the family and giving the patient continuing encouragement, in order to maintain his improvement after formal treatment is concluded.

Social phobia. Mid-way between the very specific phobias, such as phobias of insects or animals, and the diffuse collection of phobias subsumed under the term 'agoraphobia', is the social phobia. In some clients this resembles other phobias, in that the person's anxiety is quite groundless; but in others the anxiety is understandable, because the person lacks social skills, and consequently feels very uncomfortable in social situations. Another, and numerous, group of clients are so handicapped by anxiety that their skills are disrupted. For the person with basic social competence and irrational anxiety, treatment can be by desensitisation as described above, but more usually he will be encouraged to rehearse the feared situations until he feels sufficiently confident to enter them in real life. This often involves learning how to act in an appropriately assertive manner: looking people in the face, talking clearly, expressing feelings, sitting or standing in a suitable position, and so on. It is believed that being assertive counteracts anxiety in the same way as deep muscle relaxation (Wolpe and Lazarus, 1966). 'Assertiveness training' overlaps with 'personal effectiveness training' (Liberman *et al.*, 1975) and with the 'social skills training' developed by Argyle and his colleagues (Trower *et al.*, 1978). Liberman's programmes make more use of 'shaping up' the desired behaviour with consistent immediate rewards (the operant approach), and are more closely tailored to individual needs; Argyle's place greater emphasis on 'micro' behaviours, such as eye contact, and tend to follow a curriculum. The term 'social skills training' is coming to be used for combinations and variants of the three original approaches. The more detailed teaching approach is needed by those clients who lack the skills or have to relearn them. The key procedures are: breaking down the complex skill into smaller scenes or micro components of behaviour; modelling and instructions followed immediately by practice; and then feedback and reinforcement. Increasingly it is recognised that the behaviour taught during training sessions must be practised in the client's ordinary environment (Falloon *et al.*, 1977); and some workers (for example, Gambrill, 1977) introduce self-control and cognitive change procedures as another means of helping the client to generalise and maintain his new skills.

Social skills training may be provided for individual clients, with the advantage that the speed and content of the training can be adjusted to the client's requirements; or it may be provided in a group, with the advantages of modelling and support from the other members. Although there remain doubts as to the long-term effectiveness of social skills training, evidence of its usefulness with psychiatric patients is accumulating (Marzillier, 1978). Social skills training is a particularly useful addition to the social worker's repertoire.

Agoraphobia. The treatment of agoraphobia often turns out to be more complex, and treatment failures are more frequent. This diagnosis covers a wide range of different fears: of places, travel, crowds, and sometimes also of being alone or in an enclosed space. Most agoraphobic patients have multiple fears. Panic attacks, a high level of diffuse anxiety as in the anxiety state, and an admixture of depression are very common. Straightforward desensitisation to each feared situation may be tried, but it is generally agreed that flooding is the more effective approach. Behavioural treatments are usually quicker, but not conspicuously superior to other types of treatment in the long run.

In longstanding, severe cases it is necessary to make a wide-ranging assessment of the person's problems and current circumstances, and to take a history of the development of the condition. Key areas to consider include past events that might give some clues to what lies behind the fears. Often, agoraphobia begins with a severe panic attack, in which the person is afraid of fainting or dying, and this may occur soon after illness or childbirth. The fear of this happening again makes the person avoid the setting and others like it from then on. In this sort of case, an explanation of the physical aspects of the panic attack, and of the apparent basis for the development of the condition, will be helpful to the client, although rarely sufficient in itself. Another patient might give a history of being unsuccessful at school and being punished for it, so that the cluster of fears might have 'fear of failure' as a unifying theme. In this example, many behaviour therapists would decide to approach the problem as that of fear of failure rather than fear of leaving the house – but only if it can be confirmed, from the way the person feels now, that this difficulty still remains. The history of rewards for sick-role or phobic behaviour might provide clues as to what could be helping to maintain the avoidance in the here-and-now: attention and concern from other people is the most common of such factors. There have been cases in the author's experience where the wife's going out alone had upset a jealous husband, and where the patient had a long series of job-failures pre-dating the agoraphobia, yet maintained that it was 'just the agoraphobia' that prevented him from making a success of his career. The person's current circumstances must always be examined to check whether a hypothesis based on the past is still valid. In some cases, it becomes evident that some other fear, perhaps a quite realistic or at least understandable one, is playing a major part in the problem. For example, one lady lived in a block of flats with a high incidence of mugging, and had been frightened by a gang of youths. Although a housing transfer did not in itself lead to her recovery, it was only after her move that she was able to undertake a desensitisation programme which was eventually successful.

The back-up for behavioural treatment is more important for agoraphobia than for the specific phobias. It is often crucial to engage the relatives as co-therapists, and some units provide training so that they can help with treatment in an informed way (Mathews *et al.*, 1977). In such circumstances, there may be a good opportunity for social workers to learn about the behavioural approach alongside their clients.

Anxiety states. In both agoraphobia and anxiety states it may be evident that the client has one or several severe stresses to contend with, and the social worker may be able to help to mitigate these in a variety of ways. Helping the woman in the dangerous neighbourhood to find another flat is one example. Anxiety states are common in the early weeks after someone has been deserted by a spouse or lover; it may be possible to help the person to 'cool it' and take some positive action, either to resolve the situation or to begin to compensate for the loss. Marital or family discord might be eased by conjoint therapy. People with financial problems might be helped to draw up a budget and come to an arrangement with creditors.

One problem that is common among people suffering from an anxiety state is an inability to reach decisions, which may be pervasive or may centre on one particularly important choice, such as whether to leave one's partner. Social workers are particularly well equipped to help people to weigh up the alternatives open to them; and experience suggests that once having reached and implemented his decision the client feels considerably relieved. When indecisiveness is a recurrent difficulty in the person's life, repeated practice at following an ordered sequence of decision-making steps will be needed, and casework help may have to be of longer duration.

A more direct approach in the treatment of the anxiety state is a recent innovation known as 'anxiety management' (Suinn and Richardson, 1971; Meichenbaum, 1977). This approach focuses on enabling the client to develop new coping strategies, to be used whenever he feels the onset of anxiety symptoms. The client is taught how to recognise both the physiological changes and the 'self-talk' that might be producing or heightening his symptoms. He learns to relax and breathe deeply and slowly, and to make coping statements to himself. It is too early to make confident claims for this approach, but there is little doubt that it offers promise for at least some clients.

The traditional intervention for anxiety states is, of course, psychodynamic psychotherapy or casework. As we have noted earlier, it is not suitable for everyone. There is no evidence that it is better – or, for that matter, worse – than anxiety management. 'Support', and the opportunity to talk about one's troubles to a sympathetic listener, will often provide relief, although whether this relief is lasting is questionable (Marks, 1974).

But it is heartening to note that the casework treatment of 'chronic neurotic illness' (mainly a mixture of anxiety and depression) proved useful in one of the few controlled trials with a positive outcome for social work. Cooper *et al.* (1975) found that social workers attached to a general practice achieved better results in terms of both psychiatric state and social adjustment than did the control treatment. Unfortunately, the precise details of what the social workers did are not recorded.

In the following chapter we consider some less common neurotic disorders. Several of the intervention approaches suggested for phobias and anxiety states will be relevant for these too.

6

Other Neurotic Disorders

Along with some forms of depression, anxiety states and phobias, the conditions discussed in this chapter are designated 'neurotic'. This classification can be misleading: although it is generally true that the symptoms have a quality of understandability that the psychoses do not have, they can nevertheless cause great suffering and can be very resistant to treatment. Although the risk of suicide is less than for depression, it is still a danger in severe cases; patients with anorexia nervosa may die as a result of severe malnutrition; and in both anorexia nervosa and hysteria the patient can seem unaware of being psychologically disturbed, and even if not deluded, he certainly lacks the ability to make a realistic appraisal of his situation.

Obsessive–compulsive disorder

The person with this disorder feels a compulsion to perform unnecessary repetitive actions. Some of these are associated with cleanliness and tidiness, such as continual handwashing or folding of clothes; some take the form of safety checks, such as returning again and again to see that the door is locked or the gas turned off; others resemble superstitious ritual, such as rinsing the dishes a 'magic' number of times. The actions may also be internal: unproductive internal monologues and images preoccupy the person, unwanted thoughts keep recurring, sometimes in the form of alarming ideas that he might do something wicked despite himself, and some covert or overt ritual may then be undertaken to 'undo' the guilt aroused. Other patients, who do not show either obsessions or compulsions in this sense, are handicapped by excessive slowness in performing everyday activities.

Part of the usual definition of obsessive–compulsive disorder is the patient's awareness of the irrationality of his behaviour and his resistance to his compulsions and obsessions. However, some patients argue with apparent conviction that there is good reason for what they do. For example, the woman who washes her hands till they are raw may insist that she will pass on disease to her family if she fails to do this. It is hard to draw a clear dividing line between obsessive–compulsive disorder and normal experience – the child avoiding cracks in the pavement, the adult 'touching wood' for luck or trying to stop singing an old tune, the feeling that one must complete the crossword before arriving at work. However, a key difference is that the rest of us do not become severely anxious if we are prevented from doing these things, and we can if necessary control the behaviour. Midway between the two ends of the continuum is the so-called obsessional personality. This type of person is remarkable for his neatness, but the oddness and disturbing qualities are absent.

Life can become severely restricted for the person with obsessive–compulsive disorder. Friends and relatives may be unsympathetic, and their patience is sorely tried. One clever young woman, with every prospect of a successful career in publishing, lost several jobs in quick succession, because it took her five hours to get ready in the mornings; if she had been out late the night before she could not get to work till the afternoon. Her social life was equally damaged; none of her friends would have her to stay, and her flatmates could not tolerate her early rising and her monopoly of the bathroom. Obsessional thinking, although less upsetting for other people than compulsions or slowness, can prevent the person from joining in conversation or giving attention to his work. The future looks very bleak for many of these patients, and depression can arise secondary to the disorder itself.

There is also, usually, a strong admixture of anxiety. The person feels anxious if his symptomatic behaviour is prevented, and he carries it out seemingly to avoid or alleviate this anxiety. However, anxiety continues, and is exacerbated by his awareness that he is behaving abnormally.

Because of this apparent relationship between obsessive–compulsive behaviour and anxiety, psychoanalytic writers concep-

tualise these symptoms as an unconscious defence against underlying anxiety, related to fear of being unable to exert control over
the environment and to the desire to be messy, and they consider
that this disorder stems from difficulties during the so-called anal
stage of development. Little is known about causation, so that this
Freudian explanation, although without empirical backing and with
some evidence that it is incorrect, remains unchallenged by contend-
ing theories.

The prognosis for obsessive–compulsive disorder was gloomy
in most cases before the introduction of modern behavioural approaches. Without treatment, episodic improvements occur, but
with many relapses, and the illness may continue for many years.

Psychiatrists often treat obsessive–compulsive disorder with
drugs, either anti-depressants or tranquillisers. In cases where the
patient is almost totally handicapped and has suffered intolerable
distress for a long period, psychosurgery may be considered, but
this is very rare. The modern operation (which is also occasionally
performed in cases of intractable depression or anxiety of several
years' duration) is very different from the more drastic leucotomy
which produced so many cases of loss of drive or of impulse control.
The surgeon makes small lesions in precisely located areas of the
brain. This can be done under local anaesthesia and carries far fewer
dangers. Some patients show little change; others are freed of their
symptoms after one or sometimes two operations; some of these
relapse and return to their former state.

On rare occasions, a social worker may be concerned with a
patient whose psychiatrist has suggested psychosurgery. If the
social worker happens to be the team member who knows the
patient and family best, he may be asked to discuss the decision
about whether to agree to surgery. In my own experience it is helpful
to go over the details of the operation, and to visit the specialist unit,
meet the staff, and talk to other patients who have received this
treatment.

However, psychological rather than physical forms of treatment
are more usual. Perhaps the most promising development is a group
of behavioural procedures some of which parallel those used for the
treatment of phobias (Stern, 1978; Rachman, 1976). In flooding and
desensitisation the person is exposed to the situation that causes
anxiety, that is, the situation he avoids by means of his compulsive
behaviour. This may take the form of straightforwardly preventing

the handwashing, cleaning and so on (response prevention), or may be more intensive, in the sense that things around the patient are deliberately made dirty while he is forbidden or physically prevented from remedying the situation. Alternatively, the patient may be encouraged to touch dirty objects, either by way of a hierarchy from the mildly unpleasant to the very distressing (desensitisation), or by dealing with the most difficult situation right away (flooding). In all these approaches, the aim is to cause the anxiety to extinguish, and each approach seems to be successful with at least some patients. As is the case with many behavioural treatments, these approaches are not acceptable to all patients and require courage and perseverance.

For obsessional slowness, there are reports of success with some cases, using a very straightforward approach: modelling, pacing, and rewarding more rapid performance of daily tasks (for example, Bennun, 1980).

New behavioural treatments are also being developed for obsessional thinking. In 'thought-stopping', the patient learns to halt the flow of the obsessional thought pattern (Stern, 1978). Conversely, he may be instructed to keep his obsessional train of thought going, and to refrain from then carrying out his habitual internal or external putting-right procedures (Rachman, 1976). These treatments demand considerable effort on the patient's part. They have yet to be evaluated definitively, but the results so far are moderately encouraging.

The only other treatment commonly suggested is psychotherapy on psychoanalytic lines. However, most authorities would agree with Linford-Rees (1976) that psychoanalytic theory is 'of more value in explaining the psychopathology and genesis of symptoms than effecting improvement'. There is little reason to suppose that social casework on traditional lines can be useful except in offering some comfort, perhaps, and encouragement to persevere with other forms of treatment.

Social workers may contribute by enlisting support from relatives, and taking on the delicate task of getting the family involved in a programme of treatment that may require a reversal of their habitual ways of responding to the patient's problem. For example, in one programme, relatives were instructed to continue to encourage the patient to enter situations that provoked his symptoms, and to tell him to stop if he was seen to be carrying out a ritual; if this was insufficient, they were to lead him through the appropriate behaviour, calmly but firmly, and then praise him (Catts and McConaghy, 1975). As with the relatives of other types of patient, it is important not to appear to allocate blame or to condemn previous efforts to cope. In the future, behaviourally trained social workers may be able to play a part in direct treatment, especially when it takes place in the home setting.

Hysteria

There have been recent appeals for very great care in applying this diagnosis, and for greater sympathy with the sufferer. Kendell (1974) has emphasised the importance of thorough medical investigation, in order to exclude the possibility of physical disease. Hysterical symptoms can occur in association with depression or anxiety – *pace* Freud and his claim that a key feature of the disorder is *belle indifférence* – and some authorities believe that hysteria should not be regarded as an illness in its own right. The central symptom is loss of function without any identifiable physical cause: paralysis, blindness, loss of voice, lameness, fainting or fits, rather selective memory loss, the patient being apparently unaware of the 'falsity' of his disability. It is fairly rare in modern western society, and more common in other parts of the world, possibly because of differences in the culturally accepted ways of signalling mental distress. The symptoms are usually considered to be a form of symbolic solution to a psychological dilemma: in psychoanalytic terms, a way of obtaining both a primary gain (rescuing the person from some con-flict) and a secondary gain (obtaining sympathy). A simpler way of construing the person's behaviour is to see it as a desperate attempt to obtain help or make up for some lack in his life, when other avenues are not open to him.

A few psychiatrists may attempt a somewhat dramatic solution, such as performing a fake operation; but this is rarely done. Where it is considered that a traumatic experience has caused the condition, abreaction may be tried: the patient is given drugs or hypnosis, and the psychiatrist then attempts to get him to relive the trauma with its attendant emotion. Others are more concerned to make an in-depth investigation of the patient's problems, and help him to work through them and develop insight. Whether or not one of these specialised approaches is tried, it is essential to make a thorough analysis of the current situation, and to try to help with present problems, especially interpersonal ones.

Those with a behavioural background would emphasise that to try to discover whether the person is malingering or not is unnecessary (Ullman and Krasner, 1975). The focus is on a functional analysis of the person's current behaviour, finding out what purpose the disability is serving, and helping the patient to obtain the same ends by different means, while withdrawing social attention from the hysterical symptoms.

The prognosis is very variable. Hysteria can be chronic or may come and go. Occasionally, rapid and permanent cures are reported.

Amidst the argument and uncertainty about the meaning of hysteria and the likely effects of the various treatments, the social worker's tasks seem fairly clear. The social worker can play a central role in investigating current stresses and in alleviating some of these. Family interviews will be important in an effort to identify possible 'secondary' gains, as well as those problems which have brought the patient to his present predicament, and family therapy might be a means of changing the pattern. Group therapy that focuses on helping the person to learn new ways of making and maintaining relationships in an atmosphere of mutual trust and respect is another promising approach.

It may be necessary, if all else fails, to provide realistic, long-term support – in other words, befriending the patient. In one unit specialising in the treatment of hysteria, the social worker was a key figure, taking on a series of patients with hysteria who, though not 'cured', managed to cope reasonably well for most of the time. Whenever they got into difficulties, they would visit or make telephone calls and receive advice and sympathy, and it seemed they were satisfied with this and did not have to reappear with their major hysterical symptoms. This work was highly valued as a marvellous saving of doctors' time!

Psychosomatic disorders

The distinction from hysteria lies in the fact that psychosomatic disorders involve real organic pathology with presumed psychological causes. At their mildest, such disorders are familiar to everyone: diarrhoea and vomiting when feeling anxious, headaches when feeling tense, loss of appetite when feeling miserable. The list of physical conditions that may be wholly or partially caused by psychological factors is long, and constantly growing. Common examples are ulcers, digestive and respiratory complaints, and headaches, but almost every physical complaint may have some psychosomatic component. One body of evidence for this is the findings on 'life events' precipitating both psychiatric and physical illnesses (Dohrenwend and Dohrenwend, 1974).

Unless the physical illness is mild, these conditions are rarely treated by psychiatrists alone: the patient is usually seen by a physician. Thus, a discussion of psychosomatic disorder perhaps belongs more to a textbook of medical social work than to the present volume. The social worker requires the knowledge and skills to help the patient and the family to understand the psyche–soma link without causing feelings of self-blame or mutual recrimination. There may be a major role in dealing with social and interpersonal sources of stress. Just occasionally this approach seems to be a necessary and sufficient basis for a complete recovery, but we should not be over-optimistic about this: just because psychological factors are implicated, it does not always follow that the illness can be alleviated by psychological methods.

One familiar example of a psychosomatic problem is sexual dysfunction. Some social workers are now receiving training in sex therapy along the lines of Masters and Johnson (1970), and this very effective approach may be carried out in either a medical or a psychiatric setting. While it is possible for non-medical workers to recognise certain cases in which medical screening is unnecessary, most require thorough medical examination to exclude physical components (see Jehu, 1979).

Anorexia nervosa

Anorexia nervosa, though generally classified separately, is a striking example of a psychosomatic disorder. The patient is usually a teenage girl, but some males are affected, and onset is occasionally at an older age. It may continue, with periods of apparent recovery, for many years, but if it continues unabated in its severe form it can result in death. The patient starves herself, sometimes inducing vomiting; in some cases self-starvation alternates with episodes of overeating. (Some authorities consider overeating with self-induced vomiting, known as bulimia nervosa, to be a separate but related form of illness.)

Very often, anorexia nervosa begins with a slimming diet which gets out of hand, bringing serious endocrinal and medical dysfunction, as well as psychological disorder. Its psychological basis is little understood. Discord seems common in the families, along with abnormal attitudes towards food; and there is also some evidence that anorexic patients experience a fundamental disturbance of body image, having a quite unrealistic notion of their own size. (Whether these features are causes or effects of the disorder is not yet clear.) Their fear of putting on weight and/or taking food has a phobic quality, and the self-induced vomiting can resemble a compulsion.

If the anorexic patient is already severely underweight, the initial treatment will be purely medical, directed at improving the patient's physical condition. After this has succeeded to the extent that her life is no longer in danger, she may be moved to a psychiatric ward. The next step is to persuade her to eat normally.

Success has been reported with the use of behaviour modification procedures: usually depriving the patient of company, entertainment, or some valued object, and making access to these contingent upon either eating or gaining weight. Unfortunately the relapse rate appears to be high (Bhanji and Thompson, 1974). The best chance of obtaining a more lasting improvement is to work with the family as well as with the patient, so that progress achieved on the ward is maintained in the home setting. Here the social worker could play a major role. The engagement of the parents is usually not difficult (indeed they often seem to be over-involved already), but their co-operation can be threatened by a tactless suggestion of blaming the parent: for example, by hinting that the mother 'unconsciously' wants her daughter to remain a child. A main goal is to improve communication so that the patient's primitive, non-verbal messages are replaced by open discussion. Some family therapists stress the need for developing insight into the roots of the maladaptive behaviour on the part of both patient and relatives. Others concentrate on direct efforts to change family interaction in the here-and-now, favouring a directive, systems-oriented, family-therapy approach. At a more straightforward level, the family may be involved in a behavioural programme to encourage the patient to eat normally:

trying to make mealtimes into a pleasant occasion, and to avoid rewarding – perhaps by making a fuss – any reluctance to do so.

Although the evidence is sparse, it seems reasonable to suggest that family involvement can be very important in the course of anorexia nervosa and its treatment.

Hypochondriasis

In this disorder, in contrast to hysteria and psychosomatic disorder, the diagnosis rests upon a high frequency of complaints of physical illness with no physical signs. Hypochondriasis is often associated with other disorders, particularly depression. It can be construed as learned behaviour, reinforced by attention from other people, or as a face-saving way of approaching one's doctor for help with a less socially acceptable problem. Often the person is lonely and feels unloved. There is rarely any doubt of his genuine unhappiness, and 'malingering' is a totally unacceptable description; in fact, it is likely that in most cases the patient genuinely believes in the validity of his complaints.

Presenting an explanation of the disorder to patient and family has to be done with great care and sensitivity. Indeed, waiting for the patient to accept the professionals' formulation may be unrealistic. It might be better to begin with a detailed analysis of the patient's current situation, and endeavour to ensure that he gets whatever he seems to be obtaining by his hypochondriacal complaints in a more appropriate way. A consistent policy of ignoring the complaints might reduce them during the course of interviews, but this is useless unless some alternative behaviour is encouraged to take their place, and the other people around the patient join with the worker in supporting it. Change may be especially hard to achieve with some elderly patients who lead very constricted lives and have literally nothing else to talk about: they seem to use complaints about their health as a way of 'filling in' when it is their turn to say something in conversation. It may be important to look for ways of adding interest and variety to their lives, not only for the patients' sake, but for the sake of those who live with them.

There is no doubt that the patient with hypochondriasis is a very sad person. Social work help may have much to offer in order to deal directly or indirectly with his problems.

The sharing of work in relation to the disorders described in this chapter, as with depression and anxiety, requires very careful co-ordination. Views differ widely as to both the causes of the disorders and the appropriate form of treatment. Since we cannot usually point to strong evidence in favour of any single approach, each member of the team or helping network has to be willing to allow others to test out their hypotheses about what might help, as well as to offer one's own suggestions if the previous effort has failed to achieve change. Though some approaches can be tried out in parallel (for example, psychotherapy, drugs, and obtaining financial assistance), others may simply interfere with one another (for example, encouraging the person to talk freely as against a structured behavioural pro-gramme for hypochondriasis; response-prevention versus sympathy and support for obsessive–compulsive disorder). Again, a pragmatic philosophy is in order: if a powerful and energetic colleague pursues one line, trying simultaneously to follow an opposing one will bene-fit nobody, least of all the unfortunate patient! The social worker in the team has as much right to take part in discussion as anyone else, and in many situations may have more to contribute, but it is impor-tant that his comments and suggestions derive from familiarity with the recent literature as well as from his own professional experience.

7

Personality Disorders

Arguments in favour of diagnostic classification were rehearsed in the Introduction. However, 'personality disorders' are a collection of labels which, by contrast with the psychiatric illness labels, seem to serve two purposes only: they provide a form of shorthand for psychiatrists to communicate their opinions, and they provide residual ('dustbin') categories for those who feel that everyone who comes to the attention of the psychiatric services ought to be classified somehow. Not surprisingly, once it is accepted that 'personality' should be classified, there is a proliferation of different classificatory systems, each of which is further complicated by a cluster of synonyms and an overlay of euphemisms.

In this chapter I have listed the terms given in the International Classification of Diseases compiled by the World Health Organisation. Social workers (fortunately) do not need to use these terms in the course of their work, but it is useful to have some idea of their meaning – always bearing in mind that two psychiatrists using the same term might mean quite different things (Gunn and Robertson, 1976).

There is no generally accepted concept of personality disorder. One common definition is by exclusion: it is not 'illness', that is, it is not a break in the person's normal functioning. The attributes attracting the label are integral to the person. The term is used to describe certain people who are chronically unhappy, or cause difficulties for others because of relatively permanent character traits or habitual behaviour patterns that are associated with a failure to cope or to keep the rules. The traits are considered to be deviations from 'the normal', and it is largely because individual psychiatrists' ideas of 'the normal' are so variable that the label is unreliable. Priest (Priest and Steinert, 1977) highlights the problem when he mentions the danger that 'anyone more extravert than oneself is called "hysterical", or anyone less extravert is called "schizoid"'.

The International Classification of Diseases lists eight separate types of personality disorder. Two of them constitute types of 'premorbid' personality with traits that may become exaggerated and require treatment as symptoms of illness. These are the *affective personality disorder* (synonyms: cyclothymic, that is, with fluctuating mood from depressed to mildly hypomanic; depressive) and the *anankastic* (synonyms: obsessional, compulsive). It is difficult to see in what way these disorders differ from mild, chronic psychiatric illness. If the person's problems are severe enough to warrant psychiatric care the treatment is usually as for the corresponding illness.

The *schizoid personality* is withdrawn and unsociable. The *paranoid personality* shows either constant mistrust of other people or exaggerated self-importance, the key feature being excessive self-reference. It has been suggested that these may be precursors of schizophrenic-type illnesses, but evidence for this view is sparse.

The *explosive personality* is liable to sudden, uncontrollable rage (synonyms: aggressive, excessive emotional instability).

Hysterical personality is one of two types that are often singled out for discussion in textbooks (for example, Stafford-Clark and Smith, 1978), and classified as 'immaturities of personality'. (The other is 'psychopathic personality'.) The International Classification gives the following description of hysterical personality:

> shallow, labile affectivity, dependence on others, craving for appreciation and attention, suggestibility and theatricality. There is often sexual immaturity, e.g. frigidity and over-responsiveness to stimuli. Under stress hysterical symptoms (neurosis) may develop.

Another characteristic frequently associated with the hysterical personality is 'manipulative' behaviour, such as playing one member of staff off against another. For obvious reasons, people with this label are unpopular patients (the 'gross hysteric'). The treatment usually recommended is somewhat similar to that suggested for the two types of personality disorder described in detail below, the 'psychopath' and the 'inadequate'. Like them 'the hysterical personality' may be labelled 'personality disorder' without qualification – confusingly, many writers use 'personality disorder' as a euphemism for all three especially unlikeable types.

Psychopathic personality

The two types of personality disorder that appear most frequently on social workers' caseloads are the 'psychopathic' and the 'inadequate'. The term 'psychopathic' is so common that I have continued to use it here, although the International Classification of Diseases in fact uses different terms as follows:

> *Personality disorder with predominantly sociopathic or asocial manifestations*: personality disorder characterised by disregard for social obligations, lack of feeling for others, and impetuous violence or callous unconcern. There is a gross disparity between behaviour and the prevailing social norms. Behaviour is not readily modifiable by experience, including punishment. People with this personality are often affectively cold and may be abnormally aggressive or irresponsible. Their tolerance of frustration is low; they blame others or offer plausible rationalizations for the behaviour that brings them into conflict with society.

The synonyms given in the Classification are: amoral, asocial and antisocial. The term 'sociopath' and, as we have noted, the term 'personality disorder' by itself are often used as eupnemisms.

In addition to the attributes mentioned above, several other factors may play a part in the decision to diagnose someone as a psychopath (Hare and Schalling, 1978; Craft, 1966). Some authorities consider constant stimulation-seeking – doing things for 'kicks' – to be a key feature (Quay, 1965); Smith (1978) adds 'thoroughly beguiling charm'. Suggested causative factors include early-life experience, especially maternal deprivation and institutional care (Bowlby, 1951), and heredity (Storr, 1978; Eysenck, 1970).

A social history, with details of experiences thought likely to lead to the development of the 'affectionless character' or apparent psychopathy in a parent, will support the diagnosis. The social history and assessment are important in order to disentangle the personal from the social aspects of the person's behaviour. Familiarity with the norms of a particular subculture may help to clarify whether some or all of the problematic behaviour constitutes a socially approved veneer in the person's particular network: whether his aggressive behaviour, for example, is better understood in purely social rather than psychological terms. An instance of this is the teenager who acts tough and uncaring because that is the image cultivated in his gang. Smith (1978) takes this approach further, suggesting that the psychopath is not antisocial, but is an extreme manifestation of the values that western society encourages. While this view has a certain logical appeal, it offers no practical guidelines in the here-and-now.

A psychological formulation needs to take into consideration whether the problem behaviour is longstanding or habitual. Has this person a history of actions indicating lack of empathy for others, impulsive antisocial behaviour, seeming unable to learn from experience? Or is he reacting to particular circumstances, severe frustration, provocation, despair? Precisely because untruthfulness is a trait that contributes to the diagnosis of 'psychopath', the individual's own account will need to be checked, so that relatives or other professionals can confirm or refute the client's life story.

If the history tends to support the diagnosis, some psychiatrists heave a sigh of relief because they are then saved the trouble of trying to treat the untreatable! Others feel that the diagnosis ought to be avoided, because this is the one that fits the sociologists' analysis of 'labelling' best of all: the label affects our perceptions of the person, with negative consequences for his future behaviour, and the treatment he receives. Perhaps the best we can hope for is a postponement of the time when the diagnosis is written down; unfortunately, even if a psychiatrist omits the term 'psychopath', and instead gives a euphemism or, better, a careful description of the person's difficulties, whoever reads his account is quite likely to translate it back into 'psychopath'. Most social workers would try to protect the person from the harm this label can cause, but others, such as Prins (1980), have argued for its retention for a small and distinctive group of people – 'essential psychopaths' – on the grounds that they require differential treatment and management.

The closer the person resembles the 'essential psychopath', the worse the prognosis, although some authorities (for example, the International Classification of Diseases) suggest that some of the most troublesome features of the psychopath disappear with time: the person matures eventually, but more slowly than the rest of us.

There are few intervention approaches to choose from, and none that has much evidence in its favour.

Intensive group treatment is commonly recommended. In Britain, the best-known specialised settings are the psychiatric prison, Grendon Underwood, described by Gunn *et al.* (1978), and the Henderson Hospital (Whiteley, Briggs and Turner, 1972), both of which are run as therapeutic communities. The key element in their approach is the emphasis on feedback from peers in a total-living environment, where day-to-day behavioural patterns can be examined and worked on. Their success rates are difficult to determine, though there is some evidence that, while there, the residents' behaviour and attitudes do change, self-awareness is increased, and such symptoms as anxiety and depression decrease. Unfortunately, it appears that those who do best are precisely those people who show a more 'neurotic' and less 'psychopathic' picture.

The therapeutic community attempts to tackle two central attributes: inability to control impulses, and inability to 'take the role of the other'. Eysenck (1970) suggests that the psychopath is a person who is largely immune to the processes whereby most of us come to feel the stabs of conscience before or after a misdemeanour, and learn from our mistakes. If this is correct, then it follows that intensive learning experiences must be provided. The therapeutic community regime offers immediate peer group feedback, which can be very punishing or very rewarding, continuously and over a long period. This might well fit the description of an intensive learning experience. Interestingly, the therapeutic community approach has almost certainly evolved independently of the theory proposed by Eysenck, as have the communities set up by drug addicts and alcoholics, groups generally considered to contain a large proportion of psychopaths.

If the client is unwilling to enter residential treatment – and this is unfortunately the rule rather than the exception, since the psychopath does not readily volunteer for help in changing his behaviour – the social worker has few alternative measures at his disposal. Some day-centres provide a version of the therapeutic community approach. A small therapy group may be available, but it seems unlikely that this experience could be sufficiently intensive.

Some workers in the USA have begun to experiment with group-work on behavioural lines, attempting to teach the members to handle aggressive feelings in less destructive ways, and to develop empathy with others. The latter is done by role reversal, both simulated (role play), and in real life, through taking turns to perform different functions in the life of the group (Flowers, 1975).

Individual casework may be considered, although this approach seems less promising. Gunn (1978), who stresses the psychopath's vulnerability to mental illness, suggests a broad-spectrum approach, breaking the problem into small parts, tackling each part separately, and drawing on many other resources for help with work, housing, and money. It means helping the person in every way possible, and not rejecting him because of the diagnosis of psychopathy. It is sometimes suggested that a long-term experience of consistent caring may change the person's view of other people and of authority figures, may 'socialise' him, and begin to compensate for the loveless or inconsistent home he is assumed to have grown up in. Few practitioners would concur with this idealistic picture of the power of casework.

Nevertheless, there are a number of experienced workers who consider that highly skilled long-term casework may be of help. For example, Prins (1980) recommends long-term contact with one worker, and expresses some hope that if one keeps one's objectives modest, and provides a consistent, firm, but friendly relationship, the psychopath may gradually learn and change. Millard (1981a), in keeping with his formulation of the psychopath as a person whose behaviour is seriously inappropriate to its social context (frequently or persistently over time, and extensively across situations), sees the task of the social worker as 'edging people step by step' along these dimensions. In order to achieve change, considerable patience and a long series of relatively modest goals would seem essential.

Oliver (1981), in a single case study, offers some useful practical suggestions for one-to-one work with a 'personality disordered' client. Oliver placed strict limits on the amount of help offered to his client; he focused on only one problem that particularly distressed her; and he used a behavioural framework to promote impulse control. However, considerations of firmness and consistency, and even the important principle of not adding to the client's history of achieving his goals by antisocial means, have to be balanced by an awareness that there will be times when the client gets into serious trouble from which he will have to be rescued. Those habitual patterns of behaviour that have attracted the diagnosis of 'psychopathy' may continue to lead the person into distressing situations, and crises (sometimes having all the appearances of a 'contrived' or 'manipulative' crisis) are frequent. When the client's difficulties have escalated to such an extent that he is in a state of acute distress, it is possible that a crisis intervention approach could be valuable, offering rapid help and intensive casework, in the hope that at a time of upset the person will be more amenable to change (see section on crisis intervention, pp. 161–5).

Despite the unpromising label, it is probably worthwhile to make one sustained effort to help, because the psychopath and the people around him are so obviously in great need. The relatives of these clients often need assistance in their own right. Occasionally they come under a psychiatrist's care as a result of ill-treatment. Vague reassurance that their suffering will diminish as the person gets older are unlikely to be of much comfort, and we should note that authorities such as Whiteley (1975) consider that although the person may become less overtly antisocial, he will continue to behave in ways that are both self-destructive and destructive to his family. Understanding, support, and assistance in making decisions about day-to-day problems and perhaps about the long-term future, may all be of some value to the relatives: the battered wife may benefit from practical information and advice concerning her legal position and the possibility of finding alternative accommodation.

The author has attempted marital therapy with clients diagnosed as psychopathic, and has never knowingly achieved a satisfactory outcome. An example of the very limited gains is the case of a husband who left job after job, disappeared from home on frequent occasions, and slept around. He came with apparent enthusiasm to a series of conjoint sessions, in the course of which he seemed to develop some understanding of his own behaviour ('I am still like a little kid'), and communication with his wife seemed to become more open. But there was no change in his behaviour outside our sessions. Always contrite, he pleaded for sympathy in view of the enormous handicaps he suffered, top of the list being his total inability to 'really want to change'! Eventually I suggested that we were not making any more progress. The wife asked what she should do. All one can say in such circumstances is that there are two alternatives; to stay, and try to make the best of things, or to leave. I said I felt that, whatever she decided, the effort to improve their relationship had not been wasted, because knowing that one has tried seems to act as a protection against later guilt and regret. Perhaps the same factors operate for professionals after we have tried to help the most hard-to-help of all our clients.

Inadequate personality

Some of what has been said about 'psychopathy' applies here too: it is a pejorative label, with adverse consequences for the person so labelled and for professional therapeutic enthusiasm. In the International Classification of Diseases the preferred name is *asthenic personality*; and 'dependent', 'passive' and 'inadequate' are given as synonyms. 'Passive compliance', 'a weak response to the demands of daily life', 'lack of vigour' and 'little capacity for enjoyment' are cited in the definition. This diagnosis is applied even more loosely and unreliably than that of 'psychopath'. Sometimes called 'the can't cope syndrome', a history of failures, of vulnerability to minor setbacks, and a tendency to frequent the social and medical services seeking attention and assistance, seem to be the key features. People with this diagnosis make up a large proportion of psychiatrists' referrals to the social work department.

Some social workers would like to see a reduction in the number of such referrals, because they 'waste our skills', but many psychiatrists consider that social work support is the only possible way of helping. If 'support' in this context means no more than sympathetic listening and rescuing the family from recurrent crises (one might well ask 'supporting *what*?'), then it is arguable that 'support' is ineffectual, if not counterproductive, and positively unhelpful in the long run. Although admittedly we have no evidence either way, it is the author's opinion that social work skills are needed here to the full, and that the possibility of change does exist. We should not start out with the assumption that these clients will be on our caseload forever.

However, intervention does need to be quite intensive, and in order to make this possible, good caseload management is essential. It seems as though many social workers carry a large number of clients called 'inadequate', and can offer each family only irregular visits, plus emergency help from time to time. If it is decided that certain clients need someone in an 'oversight' role, then perhaps consideration ought to be given to deploying case-aides in this way, so that the trained and experienced worker can be freed to make sustained efforts with one or two of these difficult cases at a time.

At the beginning of contact, the client's lack of motivation can be a major problem. We need to consider whether the person is immobilised by anxiety, in which case we should start with a thorough, wide-ranging effort to remove as many stresses as possible, and to provide sympathy and reassurance. But just as too much anxiety prevents constructive action, so does too little; and we may have to be firm in confronting the client with realities. Perhaps the client simply cannot see any likely pay-off in attempting change; if so, it is necessary to ensure that any constructive steps are consistently rewarded. He may feel helpless, perhaps after a life history of being unable to control his environment; such clients have to be encouraged into a new series of effectiveness experiences, and this requires considerable ingenuity and perseverance on the worker's part (see pp. 42–5). The worker must be careful to avoid the appearance of expecting or rewarding 'moaning' rather than positive action.

In theory, the possibility of change ought to be assessed at the point of referral, but this is not a practicable proposition in our present state of knowledge: the possibility of change can be estimated only after a change effort has been set in motion. To begin with, it is essential to put labels aside, and to identify the excesses and deficits in the individual's repertoire. And to look beyond the individual. In psychiatric settings, it is certainly not only the poor who get labelled 'inadequate', but it is easier to cope if you have financial security. Everything is harder to cope with if you have to rear your children single-handed, have a very low income, live in an isolated and depressing tower block, and are discriminated against in the housing market. In an impossible position, even a so-called 'normal' person will become 'inadequate'.

We have to answer the question, 'can't cope with *what*?': usually, if a person is labelled 'inadequate', the list will seem formidable. The items might include housing (house-hunting, rent-paying, maintenance and repairs); housekeeping (budgeting, food preparation, housework); child-rearing (care or control); work (job-seeking, performance, work relationships); personal relationships (making and maintaining them). After drawing up the list, an agreement is reached, setting out which items will be tackled first: usually this involves a compromise between what the client finds most pressing, and what the worker knows from the literature and from experience to be most likely to alter rapidly. Having selected the target problem or a small number of problems, we have to decide on goals and tasks. What steps must be taken to modify the problem, and what would constitute an improvement in the current state of affairs?

There are a variety of behavioural procedures that have been shown to offer considerable promise in some of the problem areas mentioned above (see Gambrill, 1977 for a useful overview): specific examples include child care (McAuley and McAuley, 1977), job-seeking (Azrin, Flores and Kaplan, 1975), and social skills (Trower *et al.*, 1978). Although it is more difficult to put behavioural programmes into effect with so-called 'problem' or 'inadequate' families (McAuley and McAuley, 1980), several accounts of individual cases by behaviourally oriented social workers have shown that with a longer-than-usual time commitment and fairly intensive contact, considerable progress can be made (Bennett, 1970; Hudson, 1975b and 1976; Thomas and Carter, 1971).

A task-centred model might also be appropriate, and some of the problems might respond to marital, family or group therapy, provided the worker follows similar principles of structuring the intervention and arranging for tasks to be carried out between sessions. Step-by-step, the 'can't cope syndrome' will reduce in size, and there is a good chance that a snowballing of positive effects will occur as the person begins to feel less helpless and more competent.

There can be no doubt that there are many people we cannot help. If the sort of intervention I have described proves unsuccessful, then straightforward support and ready assistance in times of special stress may help to keep the person off the psychiatric scene. This will make demands on our patience and time, and will require un-bureaucratic flexibility.

What has been said here about intervention can apply equally to people with other forms of 'personality disorder' and also people diagnosed 'ill'. This observation illustrates the importance of looking beyond the labels to each person's specific problems. Much of this book concerns the particular difficulties of people who are grouped according to separate diagnostic labels, and people collectively designated 'the mentally disordered'. But in thinking about the so-called 'personality disorders', we are confronted most forcibly with both the commonalities and the uniqueness of all people who need social work help.

8

Problem Drinking and Drug Abuse

The abuse of alcohol, and the abuse of other drugs, have many features in common. There are serious consequences for the physical and mental health of the individual, and for the family and the rest of society as well. Often, people with these problems are classified under 'personality disorders', for understandable reasons; and it has been noted that people with severe neurotic disorders are more prone to drug or alcohol dependence than the average person (Sims, 1978). However, the evidence for a predisposing personality type is weak, the hypothesised causes of the maladaptive behaviour are diverse, and so are the responses to treatment. Social condemnation of addiction, and the association with antisocial behaviour – either as a means of obtaining supplies, or as a consequence of intoxication – combine to make provision of care and treatment, as opposed to control and punishment, an exceptionally difficult enterprise. Both groups have a raised risk of suicide (Stengel, 1973), and this is only one indicator of the immense amount of distress that is endured, sometimes behind a facade of 'lack of insight' or 'lack of motivation'.

Alcoholism and problem drinking

Definitions

The term 'alcoholic' is usually reserved for people showing particular signs and symptoms in addition to heavy alcohol intake. The key features are withdrawal symptoms after a period of abstinence (tremor and restlessness, sometimes leading to delirium tremens with severe confusion, hallucinations and the risk of convulsions); regular drinking, often beginning in the early morning; tolerance of increasingly large quantities (at a later stage tolerance again decreases); and indications of psychological as well as physical dependence.

Some authorities prefer the terms 'problem drinking', 'alcohol abuse' or 'alcohol-related problems' to cover both alcohol addiction and also heavy drinking, perhaps in occasional bouts, that has adverse consequences for the drinker and those around him. Certainly a great deal of time may be wasted at the beginning of professional intervention in trying to distinguish whether or not the person is an alcoholic, and then trying to persuade him to call himself an alcoholic. Some workers have found it possible to help the problem drinker without worrying about 'insight' in this sense (for example, Hunt and Azrin, 1973). And an 'alcoholism', i.e. an 'illness' label, can discourage the person from taking personal responsibility for change. The related message that alcoholism is an incurable disease also carries with it the notion that total and permanent abstinence is essential. This can seem very threatening, and may deter the problem drinker from seeking help; and it can cause those who do take a first drink after a period of sobriety to give up hope and continue drinking (Sobell and Sobell, 1978).

On the other hand, the term 'alcoholism' can have guilt and stigma-reducing properties and, indeed, its introduction was linked to a socio-political and humanitarian movement. Alcoholics Anonymous, which has undoubtedly made an extremely valuable contribution to the treatment of problem drinking, has found the associated beliefs that it is a disease, and that 'one drink' is the beginning of relapse, a powerful means of bolstering the determination of its members to remain sober.

Aetiology

Theories about the causes of problem drinking include such varied explanations as heredity, early childhood experience, and underlying mental disorder, especially personality disorder or depression (for a review see Royal College of Psychiatrists, 1979).

Many social workers favour the view that problem drinking is always secondary to more basic family or marital difficulties. While this is a possibility to be borne in mind, the converse can just as well be true: that the drinking problem is primary, and family dysfunction is in fact the result of stress caused to the family by the behaviour of the problem drinker. Of the many theories concerning 'the alcoholic marriage' (see Paolino and McCurdy, 1977), perhaps the most widely held is that the wife of the problem drinker is over-dominant. Orford (1975) confirmed that alcoholic husbands indeed saw themselves as 'dominated', but their wives claimed that this was not true; Chiles *et al.* (1980) concluded that 'alcoholic husbands feel submissive, but are not being forced by their wives to be so'. Cheek *et al.* (1971b) suggest that, over time, the wives of alcoholics develop a series of techniques that are intended to alter their husband's behaviour, but that may be counterproductive.

Another factor that confuses this issue is that family problems may emerge *after* the person has stopped drinking. The family of the recovered problem drinker may now feel resentment: if he can control himself after all, then he was never 'ill' in the first place, and had no right to cause them so much distress (a mechanism not uncommon in the families of other patients who have overcome their difficulties: for example, agoraphobics). Alternatively, the family may consider that now the 'illness' is over, the person should be able to make up for lost ground in double quick time; and now that he is better he should not be taking time off to see his doctor or social worker. Yet another version of the situation is that family relationship problems pre-dating the problem drinking have up till now been blamed on it; and now the family feel the lack of a 'catch-all' for their relationship or other difficulties. To sum up: it seems that in certain cases family relationship difficulties can contribute to the continuation of drinking problems, and increase the likelihood of relapse, but are rarely causal in an absolute sense.

Recognition

Problem drinking can cause many kinds of social disability, any one of which might come to the attention of a social worker. Some problem drinkers show only a somewhat reduced efficiency at work, together with lateness and brief absences; at the other end of the spectrum is the meths drinker on 'skid row'. Damage to health likewise ranges from mild impairment to fatal liver disease or irreversible brain damage.

Problem drinking tends to go unrecognised by general practitioners and social workers alike. Harwin (1979) provides a list of
common indicators that ought to alert the worker to initiate detailed
enquiries about the client's level of alcohol consumption. The indicators are social (financial problems; law-breaking; especially aggressive behaviour; work problems; frequent changes of address;
neglect of the home), familial (anxiety or depression in the spouse;
children's behaviour problems; marital discord; family violence),
psychological (anxiety or depression; overdose; sexual problems;
abuse of drugs, especially sedatives and tranquillisers), and physical
(shakiness; gastritis; burns; flu-like symptoms; obesity in young
males; accidents). If several such indicators are noted, the social
worker should ask tactfully about the client's drinking habits.
Harwin gives the weekly average amounts associated with harm:
thirty-five pints of beer, eight bottles of wine, or two bottles of
spirits. She argues that recognition of the drinking problem is essential, because it can rarely be dealt with indirectly: help with the
secondary problems that result from it, or even with stresses which
apparently play a causal role, may leave the drinking problem itself
untouched.

Treatment

Whatever the suspected original causes, the initial goal is to engage
the person in treatment. If he is strongly addicted he may be very
frightened of the process of detoxification, particularly if he has
already experienced severe withdrawal effects. It may be useful to
inform him of what to expect: he will probably receive medical care
for about a week, and medication will be given to control the unpleasant symptoms. During the 'drying out' period, efforts will be
made to improve his general health with vitamin supplements and a
planned diet.

Further help is essential. It can take many different forms. Emrick
(1975) concluded that about one-third of those treated for alcoholism remain abstinent. In general, success is associated with indicators of motivation rather than with the particular treatment
method. As yet, not all approaches have been subjected to rigorous
evaluative trials; however, it seems that with problem drinking, as
with drug abuse and personality disorder, a good outcome depends
less on the style of intervention than on the client's own determi-

nation to accept help and remain in treatment. This means that there is much to be said for giving the client the opportunity to make an informed choice, so that he can select the kind of help that best approximates to his own view of his problems and their likely solution. Insight-giving styles of therapy might appeal to the better educated and more articulate, whereas this might seem strange or very difficult to the working-class person. Alcoholics Anonymous offers group support, including round-the-clock availability of help from a fellow member, many useful commonsense suggestions, and a somewhat ritualistic – even quasi-religious – atmosphere, which seems to suit a great many problem drinkers, though not, in the author's experience, those who have become 'skid row' inhabitants. Bearing in mind the lack of firm evidence in favour of one or other of the approaches, and the need to consider each possibility in terms of how well it might suit the individual, we turn now to an overview of treatment methods, many of which can be carried out by social workers in the hospital or the community setting.

Some psychiatrists prescribe *Antabuse* (disulfiram), a drug that is incompatible with alcohol. It is taken daily in tablet form. The effects of alcohol within a few days of taking Antabuse are extremely unpleasant: usually nausea and severe malaise, but in some cases a more dangerous reaction. The patient is given a trial run of the combination. Apart from the obvious dangers inherent in this form of preventive measure and the side-effects of the drug itself, it is not uncommon for the patient to decide that taking alcohol and leaving off the tablets is a considerably more desirable proposition!

Behaviour therapy is often tried. Unfortunately the two most frequent approaches require a highly motivated client. The older method is aversion therapy: drinking alcohol is repeatedly paired with an unpleasant sensation, such as nausea or electric shock, with the goal of making the client re-experience the unpleasant feelings whenever he comes close to drinking alcohol in the future. Aversion therapy is now falling out of use, mainly because of its high relapse rate, combined with the discomfort it causes to both the client and the therapist, and the ethical problems surrounding its use. A recent variation based on similar principles is 'covert sensitisation', which involves teaching the person to associate drinking with unpleasant feelings, and resisting the impulse with pleasant ones. The client repeatedly evokes a mental image of the drinking situation, and of disagreeable stimuli and responses, such as vomiting, and then imagines himself resisting the impulse and being rewarded for it (Cautela, 1970). This approach is one of several forms of behavioural self-control treatment, and appears more promising than the therapist-delivered aversion therapy, although it is too early to make firm claims as to its long-term effectiveness. Like some of the other behavioural approaches mentioned in this book, covert sensitisation is an approach that social workers might be in a position to offer if they can obtain the necessary training.

A 'package' of behavioural methods that is of particular interest to social workers is Hunt and Azrin's (1973) 'community reinforcement' approach. The overall aim of their project was to make non-drinking more rewarding than drinking, and to help clients attain a life-style such that a return to former drinking habits would entail the loss of many forms of reinforcement. A very wide variety of services were provided. A non-drinkers' club was set up; the clients were helped to find work, and to obtain transport and a number of consumer goods, which required continuous earning in order to keep up the instalments. Help was given to reconstitute the family or resolve family or marital difficulties, and special 'alternative families' were arranged for those who had no family of their own. Many community contacts played a part in the project, not only relatives, but also friends and acquaintances. The follow-up showed this approach to be significantly more effective on several important measures, including alcohol consumption, work record, and time away from home, than was the control approach, a form of traditional group therapy. In a later paper, Azrin (1976) reported several additions which enhanced the effectiveness of the original programme: a 'buddy system' (formal arrangements for peer support), an 'early-warning system' for clients to report on imminent difficulties, group counselling, written contracts, and a reinforcement programme for taking Antabuse.

In view of the excellent results obtained by Hunt and Azrin it may seem surprising that there has not been a widespread adoption of their methods. But perhaps this is understandable: it appears to be an extremely expensive project, both in professional time (apart from the variety of treatments offered, each client was regularly visited at home), and also in terms of cash grants (the project paid first instalments on goods obtained, telephone installations, and so on). However, the general principles can be applied in other settings, and indeed can be seen at work in some of the apparently successful programmes in operation elsewhere. For example, Alcoholics Anonymous, which claims to help 75 per cent of those who join to become abstinent (Wild, 1980), has the equivalent of the 'buddy' and 'early-warning' systems, and provides social rewards for not drinking; and many hostels for recovered alcoholics offer company, food, and home comforts, so long as the person stays sober. A staff member of the London Alcoholics Recovery Project told me of his efforts to involve clients in new activities, such as going to the cinema – 'so that being sober can still mean having a good time'.

At the most general level, the aim of making abstinence more rewarding than drinking should guide our planning. This is particularly important for those alcoholics who belong to an alcoholic subculture and have no other ties: no job, no family, no non-alcoholic friends. If they give up drinking, they have much to lose and little to gain in the short term, and it is the short-term consequences that are most powerful in maintaining the behaviour of most people with addictions. A major challenge to our skills and ingenuity is to find a way of reversing the contingencies.

Recent evidence (Sobell and Sobell, 1978) suggests that we should always begin with a detailed functional analysis of the individual's drinking pattern. This means exploring tie precipitants of problem drinking and the purposes that drinking seems to serve for each individual. These can vary widely, but frequently include some of the following: dealing with anxiety, staving off depression, helping one to sleep, as a pain-killer, to calm oneself after an argument, and the social rewards of drinking. In the case of people who have been heavy drinkers for many years, the role of such factors may have become obscure, and the main precipitant may now be simply a craving sensation. Once identified, each contributing problem will require separate attention. For example, inability to resist social pressure may respond to assertiveness training; anxiety and depression to the treatments appropriate for these disorders; and so on. A related approach is to analyse the chain of thoughts, feelings and actions that culminate in drinking alcohol, and to assist the client to become fully aware of this progression, and to devise strategies for interrupting the chain before he reaches the point of no return. Covert sensitisation, described above, provides one such strategy; others might include avoiding certain acquaintances or places, entering upon different activities, or relaxing whenever the craving sensation appears.

Recently, some behaviourally oriented workers have begun to advocate moderate drinking as a goal, rather than total abstinence (for example, Strickler *et al.*, 1976; Sobell *et al.*, 1972). In these programmes, the client is given instruction on what and when he should drink, and on drinking 'style' and suitable quantity. This is accompanied by training based on behavioural principles, to analyse his drinking patterns as described above, to judge the level of alcohol in the blood, and to substitute activities incompatible with drinking, such as deep muscle relaxation. Spouses are also involved in these programmes, in order to support the client's efforts as well as to reduce any counterproductive interaction.

'Controlled drinking' may be a more attractive goal if the client moves in circles for whom social drinking is the main leisure activity; and it is certainly a less threatening prospect than permanent abstinence. A great deal of further research is required before this can be confidently recommended; however, for some clients it might be worth trying, with the proviso that the goal of total abstinence may have to be substituted if the attempt fails.

Several of the programmes already mentioned have included some form of *group therapy*. This is a very common approach, either by itself or as an adjunct to individual treatment, and our knowledge of the power of group processes, and the generally favourable results of group therapy with a variety of conditions (Bednar and Lawlis, 1971), provide a strong rationale for offering group support to problem drinkers. However, its effectiveness as a sole treatment for alcoholism has not been established (Whiteley and Gordon, 1979). One possible reason is that so much of the problem behaviour is under the control of circumstances quite remote from the group setting: in the community, at work, or at home.

Working with the spouse

The spouse of the problem drinker has already been mentioned as a possible source of help in overcoming the drinking problem, and the marital relationship as one possible source of stress that could precipitate drinking. Often it is the spouse who comes for professional help rather than the person with the drinking problem. Meyer (1978) offers suggestions as to how the spouse might be able to improve the chances of his or her partner seeking help. For example, she proposes that the partner should make no attempt to shield the problem drinker from the consequences of heavy drinking. There are times, when the person is sober, when a good opportunity occurs (but is often missed) to talk seriously, but with affection and compassion, about the difficulties that are causing damage to the relationship. These suggestions have received empirical support in the findings of Schaffer and Tyler (1979): alcoholic husbands were more likely to remain sober if their wives were able to communicate their feelings of distress and frustration in a non-threatening manner.

However, it will often be necessary to try to give assistance to the spouses alone. Sympathetic listening may provide some temporary relief, but they will also require help in coping on a day-to-day basis, to alleviate their difficulties even if only in small ways, and to make longer-term decisions for themselves and their children. Their confusion and fear prevent them from taking a cool look at their situation, and lack of financial resources makes separation extremely difficult for many wives. Some spouses will eventually decide that they can stand no more. The husband or wife may then become motivated to attempt to change; others will deteriorate even further when left on their own.

Skid row

There will remain after all our efforts many people who continue to abuse alcohol, and of these, some will end on 'skid row'. Failure to provide these people with even the basic necessities of life is a matter of very grave concern. Provision is largely left to voluntary agencies with few resources. These agencies require the wherewithal to arrange health care and to give their clients a reasonable diet and a comfortable bed. It is often as a result of relationships formed with workers in such agencies that clients begin to feel sufficient trust and hope for the future, to say they are ready to 'take the cure'; and it is a sad reflection on our services that red tape and bureaucratic delays can then intervene, and the person's motivation seeps away again before he can be admitted for medical care.

The police, the lodging houses for homeless single people, and the social security department are other agencies with whom the social worker might usefully liaise. All these organisations have a wide area of discretion as to how they respond to the person with a drinking problem. If the psychiatric services are willing to share their knowledge and experience, and to offer help as and when it is needed, a more effective caring network can be made available (Spratley, 1978).

Drug abuse

Drug abuse refers to drug-taking that constitutes problem behaviour, whether or not the person becomes dependent.

Drug abuse shows many similarities to alcohol abuse, in both its symptoms and its effects. It can be construed in behavioural terms, emphasising the purposes it seems to serve for the individual and the chain of events that lead to taking the drug, and a broader approach stresses the need for an alternative life-style to compete with the person's current situation.

As with problem drinkers, there are solitary drug-abusers and also a drug subculture. There are also 'fashions' in drug abuse, so that a run on glue-sniffing, for example, may sweep one district or age-group, to be replaced by petrol-sniffing the following year. (But it is worth noting that many young people seem to drift in and out of a drug subculture without permanent harm.)

There are a great variety of possible drugs of abuse, ranging from the generally illegal drugs such as heroin, cocaine, morphine and LSD, to the medically prescribed, such as amphetamines and barbiturates.

The common drugs of abuse fall into three major groups: sedative, stimulant and hallucinogenic (Willis, 1976), but it should be remembered that some people take several types of drug, particularly those who move in drug-taking circles.

Heroin and morphine are strongly addictive drugs of the sedative–analgesic type. While the person is on the drug, there are few outward signs, except for marks on the arms and legs where he has injected himself. At first these drugs are taken for the sense of euphoria (the 'buzz'), but quite soon their main value seems to be in reducing the unpleasant withdrawal effects, which include restlessness, irritability, stomach cramps and digestive upsets. There are serious health risks, especially from infection from the syringe used for injections and from the effects of malnutrition and self-neglect.

Hypno-sedative drugs include barbiturates, which may have been

prescribed for insomnia. Users may suffer from chronic intoxication, with slurred speech, drowsiness, and confusion. Withdrawal
can cause delirium, fits, severe restlessness. Those addicted to barbiturates include many more women than the other groups, and this
form of drug abuse is at least as prevalent among solitary drug-users
as in drug subcultures.

The stimulants are another group of drugs which have often been
medically prescribed, particularly for women who wish to lose
weight. Amphetamines are the most common. When they are left
off, the person feels lethargic and miserable; but they can cause
restlessness, irritability, and, if large amounts are taken, psychosis
closely resembling acute schizophrenia.

The third main group are the hallucinogenic drugs. LSD is unpredictable in its effects: the LSD 'trip' can be intensely pleasurable,
producing a dramatic and beautiful vision of the world and feelings
of power or new creativity, but it can also cause severe depression or
panic, and psychosis, and these effects may last or recur. Some
people have died during a bad 'trip'. LSD does not cause physical
dependence, but is nonetheless one of the most dangerous of drugs
of abuse.

Cannabis can have similarly agreeable, but much milder, effects: a
feeling of well-being, a delightfully altered perception of the world.
But as with LSD, this can vary according to the individual and the
occasion. There seems to be little evidence that cannabis causes
untoward effects or induces dependence (Stafford-Clark and Smith,
1978).

Recognising that a drug problem exists is not always easy when
the person is addicted to a medically prescribed drug. However,
these clients are more likely to co-operate in treatment than the
drug-culture members discussed later; and those who have been on
amphetamines may respond to social support, and treatment for
their depression on an out-patient basis. Those on barbiturates will
probably require a brief hospital stay, during which the drug will be
withdrawn gradually.

The medical treatment for dependency on heroin and other drugs
in this group consists of medication to combat the severe and sometimes dangerous withdrawal effects. Some patients are given a substitute drug: best known is the prescription of methadone. In
Britain, certain doctors are licensed to prescribe the person's drug of
addiction; this may then be reduced gradually or at least rationed,

and the clinic contacts are used to try to motivate the person towards an attempt to 'kick the habit'. As is the case for drinking problems, a great deal of help is required in addition to detoxification.

There have been few controlled studies to evaluate the effects of the different treatment approaches. Many behavioural writers propose the same methods as those outlined in the section on problem drinking (see also Gambrill, 1977). A few interesting single case studies have been published, and might suggest possible ways of proceeding, although they do not constitute a basis for optimistic adoption of their methods. One innovative example concerns a woman who applied an operant-conditioning approach to her own behaviour, with powerful motivation supplied by her therapist: with her written agreement he held several cheques signed by her and made out to the Ku Klux Klan, of which she strongly disapproved, on the understanding that if she again took drugs he would send the cheques off (Boudin, 1972). Without wanting to minimise the success achieved in this case, one is left wondering how many clients would have the motivation or self-confidence to agree to such a plan, and further, whether all of them could be trusted to report back as honestly as this woman apparently did.

Drug subcultures can be especially powerful. Some social workers, operating from shop-front or street agencies, have found it possible to 'get alongside' young people who are involved. By a slow process of earning their trust, and perhaps also by acting as a model who is seen to have some similarities with the client, they have sometimes been able to encourage a change of attitude, and to 'seize the moment' to facilitate an attempt to seek formal help. For those clients who become willing to give up the double attachment of the drugs and the drug world – and this often occurs at a time of crisis, such as a court appearance or a hospital admission – it is important to give a message of concern without condemnation, and to make an offer of immediate help.

Because of the power of the ties binding many of these clients, the most promising form of help appears to be referral to a facility that offers intensive group experience in a residential setting. Apart from providing direct treatment, these communities allow the client to find a place in an alternative miniature society, with different norms, but with some of the same satisfactions of 'belonging', plus the company of similar people. Many of these communities are run by ex-addicts, whose ability both to empathise and to model an alternative way of life are accompanied by a right to tough talking, which can only be claimed by someone who has personally overcome the difficulties the client is experiencing.

The success rate achieved by such communities is hard to judge. The drop-out rate is high, and it certainly seems as though it is only the client who is desperate to change who will stay the course. Confrontation, insight-giving, and the obligation to take responsibility, are the keynotes of these regimes. In behavioural terms, they appear to make extensive use of punishment rather than positive reinforcement. But some clients will benefit, and benefit permanently (Whiteley and Gordon, 1979).

In our present ignorance regarding effective forms of intervention, and since a few clients will be successful in any intensive change programme, clients should be supported and actively encouraged to try whatever type of treatment is available and acceptable. And if the client fails on the first attempt, this is not a reason for assuming that the second or third attempt will not be successful.

This said, drug-dependent clients are another group that includes many 'therapeutic failures', who nevertheless have some needs that we can meet. There is a danger with these clients, as with so many others, that the medical and social services will do nothing, simply because they cannot do everything.

9

Organic Disorders with Special Reference to the Elderly

It is impossible to discuss the organic psychiatric syndromes without frequent reference to the elderly. This chapter begins, therefore, with an overview of old age and mental disorder, as a necessary backdrop to our main topic. The organic psychiatric syndromes (synonyms: organic brain syndromes, acute and chronic brain failure, organic psychoses) are those disorders in which psychological disturbance is due to a definite, recognisable physical cause. The disruption in brain function that leads to psychological disturbance can be either temporary (acute), or permanent, and often progressive (chronic). To describe all types of organic disorder would be inappropriate in a textbook for social workers, and only the more common conditions are included. Epilepsy, which is generally the province of the neurologist rather than the psychiatrist, is briefly discussed in a separate section at the end.

Old age and mental disorder

The high rate of organic psychiatric syndromes among old people tends to overshadow the equally important fact that other forms of psychiatric disorder affect the elderly as they do the rest of us, and respond to treatment in exactly the same way.

Depressive illness is not only more common with increasing age, it also carries a higher risk of suicide (Arie, 1979). There is often severe agitation, and in some cases symptoms that can be mistaken for dementia. *Depressive pseudo-dementia* is a recognised syndrome which responds to anti-depressive treatment. *Hypomania*, too, is not uncommon, and is as treatable in the elderly as it is in younger people.

Another psychotic illness that requires special mention is *late paraphrenia*. Usually considered, and treated, as a form of schizophrenia, paraphrenia is diagnosed on the basis of prominent delusions, usually of persecution, which are embedded in a complex system of beliefs. Thus the person may believe he is being persecuted by large organisations which communicate with one another in special ways and have elaborate plans to bring about his downfall. In contrast to other forms of schizophrenia, in paraphrenia there are few other symptoms (except auditory hallucinations in some cases). The person is often able to manage his life and appears normal, until he begins to talk about his delusional system or to make accusations which upset or inconvenience other people.

Where medical treatment fails to dispel the psychotic symptoms, our 'target system' may have to be the people who complain of the patient's behaviour, reassuring them and trying to gain their sympathy and understanding.

Neurotic disorders are common, especially *depression*. This is hardly surprising when we consider the many losses and life changes to which old people are subject: bereavement, often multiple; loss of role as worker; reduction in income; loss of one's home and one's privacy and independence; and failure of physical functions such as hearing, eyesight and mobility. Add to these the undoubted lessening of respect for older people in our society, and the isolation that results from the geographical dispersal of the extended family, and we have a catalogue of stress and loss of support that makes the increased rates of depression and suicide readily understandable. It is difficult, indeed, to distinguish between depression as an illness requiring medical intervention, and understandable unhappiness proportionate to the person's situation, but it is important to try to do so. Willis (1974) warns against the danger of supposing that an individual is a lonely old person when in fact he is a lonely, depressed old person.

With ageing there is also an increase in problems likely to cause *anxiety*: living alone without the means of calling for help in case of illness or accident; financial worry; fear of mugging or burglary; fear of being 'put away'. Often, attitudes belonging to an earlier social climate play a part in exacerbating anxiety. For example, poverty still means fear of the workhouse for many old people. Respectability and independence (not that these values are the exclusive province of the elderly!) are often of overwhelming significance, in part perhaps because other goals, such as success in work or social life, can no longer be actively pursued.

All of these, and problems that are problems for everyone – loneliness, family discord, poverty and poor housing – take their toll in this as in every other age-group.

Social casework can be effective in relieving these problems to at least some degree (Goldberg *et al.*, 1970). The elderly can also benefit from groupwork run on exactly the same lines as for younger clients: problem-solving, behavioural (social skills training), or more traditional social groupwork (Toseland and Rose, 1978).

Sadly, many social workers still take the attitude that there is little need for skilled – that is, individually tailored and informed – social work, and that all the elderly need is the routine provision of concrete services.

Finally, and perhaps most important of all, doctors and social workers alike should not forget the high rate of *normality* in old age. Deafness, poor eyesight, tremor, and a general slowing down, are among the many factors that can lead to a mislabelling of the elderly person. One old lady was almost taken to a psychiatric ward, because she was found hammering on the door of a shop an hour before opening time – it turned out that her clock (her son's responsibility) was one hour fast. No one had given her the chance to give her version of what was happening. Another lady was diagnosed as paraphrenic, because she complained of being followed about and abused by a gang. Her social worker accompanied her on a shopping expedition (keeping at a distance) and, sure enough, a group of boys marched after her, calling her names like 'witch' and worse!

Confusional states (synonyms: acute organic brain syndrome, brain failure, delirium, acute cerebral dysfunction)

Confusional states are extremely common, and they can occur at any age. In younger people, they are most likely to develop in association with acute physical illness, or after an operation. When seen in the community, the sufferer is usually an elderly person with a very mild infection. Onset can be sudden. The confusional state is generally short-lived, but there is considerable variation in both duration and severity, depending on the course of the underlying condition. The person's mental state fluctuates, usually being more disturbed in the evening.

The central feature is impairment in the level of consciousness. This causes a reduction in the person's ability to grasp and retain information, which shows itself in a variety of ways, especially disorientation (not knowing where one is or what day it is, not recognising people or following what they say), and inability to concentrate on any one thing at a time. The sufferer may seem ill-tempered and restless, and is perplexed and usually very frightened. Sometimes more dramatic symptoms appear, some of them probably stemming from the person's inability to comprehend his situation, and his consequent fear: illusions (mistaking the identity of people or things), delusions of persecution, and extremes of anger or panic. However, *any* psychiatric symptom can occur in a confusional state.

Confusional states accompany general metabolic or toxic changes in the body. Willis (1976) estimates that there are some sixty different physical causes. These include chest and urinary infections; heart, liver or kidney failure; poisoning due to drugs or alcohol; and local brain damage from any cause, such as head injury or stroke. One familiar type is delirium tremens (DTs). This occurs after withdrawal of a drug of addiction. Though it is best known in association with alcoholism, it also follows withdrawal of several other drugs, including barbiturates. Common causes of confusional states among the elderly are mild infections, constipation, the effects of malnutrition, and hypothermia due to inadequate heating.

Intervention

The key intervention is of course medical investigation and treatment of the underlying condition. The confusional state will then usually clear quickly, but in some cases – especially if the patient is elderly and has a mild pre-existing memory impairment – it may take many weeks to improve. If this is the situation, it is extremely important that no precipitate action be taken, on the assumption that the person will require permanent hospital care. The flat, or place in an old people's home, must be kept on, and the pets must be cared for, so that when the person recovers he is not faced with irrevocable and unnecessary losses.

All who have contact with the elderly in the community need to be able to recognise a confusional state, so that they can call in medical advice as a matter of urgency. The most important clue is a recent change in the person's mental state. Other information that may be useful to the doctor in his investigations includes such details as an unexplained fall, an accident, suspected failure to take medication, misuse of drugs, or any signs of self-neglect.

When he recovers, the patient may still be distressed by vague memories of preceding events. It is essential to reassure him that this is not the beginning of a dementing process. And the family, equally, may need this help. They may well have jumped to the conclusion that the person has 'gone off his head', and they may be living in fear of a repetition. Where a vulnerable elderly person is concerned, a conference of family members and other helpers is useful, in order to work out strategies to prevent a recurrence of the crisis. Close attention will have to be paid to warmth, diet, and future surveillance. The social services or a voluntary agency may be involved, to assist with practical needs, and to provide regular visiting to ensure that the person's health does not deteriorate again without prompt medical attention.

Chronic organic disorders of the elderly: senile dementia and multi-infarct (arteriosclerotic) dementia

Dementia has been described as 'a remorseless enemy of the natural dignity of man' (Stafford-Clark and Smith, 1978). The term 'dementia' refers to a cluster of symptoms, irreversible except in certain very rare conditions, and occurring in clear consciousness. The most prominent symptoms are intellectual deterioration and memory impairment, and in most cases they are accompanied by emotional lability, loss of drive, and a lowering of standards of behaviour.

Estimates of prevalence among the elderly range from one in ten of those over sixty-five, to one in five of those over eighty. While noting that dementia is the most frequent reason for hospital care of patients over seventy, we should bear in mind that other psychiatric disorders are also common in old people, and that most people reach the end of their lives without suffering from dementia. Nevertheless, dementia in the elderly might well be designated the major psychiatric problem of our time, and as life expectation increases, this problem will increase in parallel.

The two most familiar disorders causing dementia are senile and multi-infarct dementia, and are diseases of the elderly. Multi-infarct (arteriosclerotic) dementia is caused by numerous small infarcts, and senile dementia by a more general widespread wasting of the brain. Multi-infarct dementia may occur in someone who has shown other evidence of vascular accidents (strokes), and is usually less devastating in its effects on personality, at least in the early stages. However, the end result is the same for both types of dementia. The effects of certain drugs on multi-infarct dementia are currently being investigated, but with little positive evidence so far, and there is no known drug treatment for senile dementia. The two disorders are difficult to distinguish from one another, and the social worker's approach to helping will be guided by the severity of the person's handicap, rather than by the specific diagnostic category.

Memory deterioration (in the short term at first) is usually the initial impairment. One lady, who was staying with her niece in a strange town, went out for a walk and lost her way. She called in at an office, and very sensibly asked if she might consult a telephone directory in order to look up her niece's address, which she had forgotten. Then she found she could not recall her niece's married name. This illustrates how memory loss can be quite severe before other intellectual functions are affected.

Memory impairment can have a number of distressing consequences, not only for the patient, but for other people around him. For example, he may put his money, key or pension book in a safe place, but the place is then forgotten and he insists that they have been stolen, and becomes paranoid towards family, neighbours or helpers. Another extremely trying feature is the tendency to ask the same question over and over again, since the reply is forgotten immediately it is given.

As the dementing process continues, thinking becomes less subtle and less logical. There is disorientation as to place, time and person, leading to wandering. The emotions become shallow and labile, disproportionate distress giving way abruptly to inappropriate gaiety. Later, the person may become aggressive, dirty, and may develop odd habits like packing suitcases with unsuitable objects, hoarding things, talking to invisible people and 'living in the past'. In a few especially tragic cases, the person may commit illegal actions, such as acts of sexual indecency or stealing from shops. One of the saddest features is the fact that the early stages of dementia may be accompanied by awareness of deterioration and consequent severe anxiety and depression.

Intervention

There are no satisfactory answers as to how to go about helping the person with early dementia. We need to be aware of the person's sensitivities – not driving him into corners and drawing attention to his memory defects. Nevertheless, it is helpful to provide, repeatedly but tactfully, the information he is most prone to forgetting, such as the day, the time, and the names of people and places. Obviously, a social worker would avoid expressions of surprise or irritation, but it is all too easy to slip into the opposite type of unkindness, treating the person as far less intelligent than he actually is. A person with a poor memory does not have to forfeit the courtesies of ordinary adult communication, and even those who are quite badly affected can join in conversation, and appreciate being asked for help or advice, if only in small everyday matters like cooking or clothes. A well-run social club or day-centre, where the members are not babied and are given opportunities to socialise and to contribute to the group's activities, can do much to bolster self-esteem and ward off depression.

At this stage the doctor or social worker may be especially concerned with the question of how much to tell the patient and his family about what is wrong. Priest (Priest and Steinert, 1977) suggests the analogy with a serious illness like cancer, and proposes that they be given the opportunity to ask questions and receive information at their own speed, with the option of curtailing the discussion whenever they wish. It is not just a matter of providing information, of course: it is also essential to 'stay with' the person who reacts with grief, despair, anger or fear.

At times, a son or daughter, or a spouse, will express quite unrealistic hopes of a cure and a return to normality. If often seems that this is whistling in the dark, and the relative knows the truth and is merely repeating such hopes in a desperate attempt to comfort himself. It is the right of the person who is being 'bereaved' in this manner to take his own time to come to terms with the real situation. And in these circumstances, acting 'as if' can itself be beneficial for the patient if it means continued respect and care, rather than despair and possibly rejection.

Another topic that can arise at this time is the future care of the patient. Many express fear of being 'put away', and the relatives may dread the day when they can no longer cope. It is quite realistic to point out that no one can predict the future – many patients do not in fact live long enough to experience the worst ravages of a dementing disorder; and it is important to add the assurance that the person will be given whatever form of care is judged to be in his best interests, whether that is at home, or in a hospital, or something in-between.

As the disorder progresses, communication with the dementing person becomes increasingly difficult. The social worker will need to give constant reminders of who he is, and why he is there, and when he will call again. Written reminders, large and clear, are helpful to many of these clients. It is important to speak slowly, and to give time for each statement or question to be registered, and for the client to organise his response – anxiety tends to increase confusion and incoherence. Gray and Isaacs (1979) suggest that the worker should show particular interest when the person talks rationally, and should try to 'encourage a lucid interval' by mentioning some aspect of the past that the client can recall with pleasure. People whose speech is badly affected are often able to express themselves non-verbally – they may be able to show their uncertainty, agitation or pleasure through varying their grip on the hand.

On the practical side, there are a number of measures that might alleviate some of the problems of the dementing patient. Chief among these is medical intervention: treating physical illness that may be contributing to incontinence, and medication for anxiety, depression and agitation. At least during the initial phase, the effects of poor memory can to some degree be combated by simple expedients, such as keeping a notebook and a memo board, and a prominently displayed calendar showing the day and the date; and making sure that the patient's name and address are in handbag or pocket, so that getting lost is less traumatic than it would otherwise be. Opportunity for acitivity and variety are considered to be beneficial by most authorities. This may have little or no effect on intellectual impairment, but at least it will increase the person's sense of well-being, and make the most of his remaining capacities. Seligman (1975) points out that the elderly are often treated in ways that seem highly likely to lead to a state of learned helplessness. With this in mind we ought to be imaginative in attempting to increase rather than narrow the person's sphere of control. One particularly 'helpless' lady proved very skilled at entertaining a neighbour's two-year-old; another was able to take charge of the family breakfast.

In recent years, more systematic techniques have begun to be evaluated. Engagement in activities can be increased by methods that could be used at home, in a day-centre or residential home, or in groupwork. For example, research by the Wessex Health Care Evaluation team has demonstrated the value of such simple measures as making recreational materials readily available, and giving attention contingent upon activity instead of showing interest mainly when the person is not participating (Jenkins *et al.*, 1977; Powell *et al.*, 1979). Similarly, McClannahan and Risley (1975) showed that placing materials in the clients' hands, and prompting them to use them, led to a significant rise in the level of participation. The Wessex team also established that people's expressed attitudes to activities did not predict what they actually did when offered the opportunity to take part.

An interesting groupwork experiment (Linsk, Howe and Pinkston, 1975) showed that active questioning, and consistent reinforcement for contributing to the discussion, resulted not only in an increase in appropriate talk in the group, but also in willingness to attend. This was in contrast to the results obtained with a less structured, more *laissez-faire* type of leadership.

Another method that is currently being evaluated is 'reality orientation therapy'. This is a time-consuming approach which tries to modify the key symptoms of dementia directly. It seems to require great patience and perseverance from the worker, but the results to date suggest that it has some success in helping patients to orient themselves with regards to time, place, and people's names (Greene *et al.*, 1979; Woods, 1979). The clients are given intensive practice, and consistent, immediate reinforcement for answering questions correctly and making appropriate remarks. As might be expected, the results are better for the less severely demented, and generalisation to different situations remains problematic. All these approaches might be relevant for social workers concerned with clients suffering from dementia.

Since there is evidence that a change of environment can make matters worse, all manner of measures to delay or prevent removal from home must be considered, measures focusing as much on the family's as on the patient's well-being. The burden on the family can be immense, surpassing even that experienced by the relatives of the chronic schizophrenic patient (Grad and Sainsbury, 1968). It is essential to try to alleviate the strain at an early stage, rather than allow the home situation to deteriorate to a crisis point, with the family totally exhausted and angrily refusing to carry on.

Practical forms of help are less difficult to envisage than they are to obtain. They include relief for the family, such as sitters for a few hours or holiday respite for a period of weeks, laundry services, and day-care if only for a day or so a week.

The family will also appreciate straightforward advice about day-to-day problems. They could be encouraged to experiment with ways of reducing pressure on the patient, of rewarding rational talk, of finding simple tasks for him to do – another example of the relative as therapist. Artificial and mechanical as this suggestion might seem, it does appear that the relative in this role is more tolerant and less distressed, though we do sometimes need to emphasise that 'being a therapist' does not mean infantilising the elderly person.

Less obvious, but just as important, is help with the feelings of bewilderment, annoyance and grief that most relatives experience. First and foremost, we ought to express appreciation for the burden they carry. They may need help to understand the patient's behaviour, so that they can begin to recognise and accept those features that are 'part of the illness', rather than castigating themselves or the patient. Especially sad are those cases where a spouse has to watch his partner deteriorating; often he will react like someone who has been bereaved. The support of a relatives' group, and the practical advice and help that relatives can provide for one another, could be useful; but when the elderly person is being cared for at home it may be difficult for the relative to attend, even if transport is laid on. And it is quite understandable that many relatives prefer to take the opportunity to do something else on the rare occasion when they are free to leave the house for a while!

If there comes a time when the family feel they can no longer continue to care for the dementing person, they may need considerable casework help before they can reach a decision. Although it is a decision that cannot be made for them, the social worker can at least ensure that they have had the opportunity to examine all available alternatives, and that they will be able to look back on their decision with the knowledge that it was not taken hastily or in ignorance. Even so, after suffering the burden of caring for the patient at home, these relatives will often feel great guilt after they have allowed him to be 'put away'. Support and reassurance at this stage may make it possible for them to continue to visit and to care, instead of avoiding the person because seeing him reawakens their guilt.

Groups for relatives visiting the old people's home or the hospital can also provide support. If the meetings have a 'social' element, they may enable the members to make friends, and the journey and the sometimes trying conversation with the elderly person will seem the more worthwhile.

While relatives' associations on behalf of younger patients are growing more influential, similar groups for the relatives of psychogeriatric patients are rarer. They can be of great value in working for proper standards of care in our hospitals and homes.

Chronic organic disorders beginning prior to old age (the pre-senile dementias)

These are much rarer than the senile and multi-infarct forms. They resemble them in symptomatology and course, but are very much harder for the family members to accept, and even experienced professional workers feel deeply distressed and impotent in their wake. Only the most common of these disorders are discussed here, with some of their distinguishing features.

Alzheimer's Disease and Pick's Disease

These disorders usually begin in late middle age. Little is known about their aetiology, and they closely resemble senile dementia in symptoms and course.

Korsakoff's syndrome (Korsakoff's psychosis, the dysmnesic syndrome)

The main features of Korsakoff's psychosis are severe impairment of short-term memory, attempts to fill the gaps with plausible invented details (confabulation), and disorientation in time. General intelligence seems not to be affected, and the person may well be aware of his difficulty, although some patients appear emotionally 'flat', or inappropriately cheerful.

The main cause is a vitamin deficiency, usually associated with heavy alcohol intake over a long period, and the disorder is most frequently met with in middle-aged alcoholics. Other causes are infections such as encephalitis, tumours, or brain injury.

In a small minority of cases involving vitamin deficiency there is some hope of arresting the course of disorder, but even in these the damage already suffered is permanent. However, the fact that some cases of chronic organic disorder are treatable means that urgent medical investigation is a vital first step in dealing with any case of dementia.

Huntington's Chorea

This usually begins in early middle age with symptoms of clumsiness, restlessness and often depression. 'Chorea' refers to the involuntary jerking movements, and these, combined with other neurological impairment, eventually lead to physical disability. This is accompanied by the full range of symptoms of dementia. Behaviour disturbance is common, and in many cases a paranoid psychosis also develops, indistinguishable from schizophrenia. The patient usually dies within about fifteen years from the time of diagnosis.

Huntington's Chorea is a hereditary disease, and exact predictions can be made concerning the pattern of inheritance. There is a fifty–fifty chance that any child of a parent with the disorder will develop it. Since it does not normally show itself until after the time when most people become parents, the person at risk, if he is ignorant of the facts, may not be able to avoid passing it on to the next generation. Tragically, those who decide to remain childless cannot even console themselves with the prospect of adopting children, since the uncertainty of their own future health, and the likelihood of life-long anxiety about themselves and their relatives, will militate against their being accepted as adopters.

Not surprisingly, members of Huntington's families suffer untold misery, and the rates of suicide, alcoholism and depression are high. Some find a glimmer of hope in the fact that research is proceeding rapidly, expressing confidence that a cure may be discovered. Many try to cope by denying the facts, or adopting an inaccurate though consoling view of the disorder – for example, that it always misses a generation, or that inheritance is linked to sex of the parent or child.

Some social workers have specialised in work with these families, offering a combination of support, practical help, and counselling (Martindale and Bottomley, 1980; Ramsay, 1976). In both Britain and the USA there are specialised voluntary associations which offer information, advice and support.

Before ending this overview of chronic organic disorders, it should be mentioned that there are a variety of very rare disorders, and other conditions such as head injuries, tumours and certain endocrine and metabolic diseases, that can cause dementia and/or other psychiatric symptoms. (Willis (1976) is a useful reference text.)

Intervention

The role for social work, as in cases of organic disorder in elderly clients, lies in offering support to the patient, information and casework to the family, and practical services to improve the situation at home, so that the patient can remain there for as long as possible.

One problem area that is especially poignant is the question of separation when one of a married couple is affected. When onset is gradual, the relationship may be particularly difficult. One wife said she could not bear it 'when he seems normal', and longed for the time when her husband would be 'finally changed from what he was'. Another young woman found it impossible to resist clandestine evenings out, and eventually began an affair, which was blighted by her feelings of guilt, and her fear of what people would think of her for failing to remain loyal to her severely demented husband.

Sexual problems can cause misery to both partners – for example, the patient may continue to show sexual desire, while the partner feels repelled. In cases like these, the spouse may feel very alone and unable to discuss the problem with anyone. A great deal of gentle probing and 'giving permission' will be necessary before the problem can be openly acknowledged. In the author's experience, it is an exceptionally difficult personal challenge to offer this kind of help, and the worker may be as prone to avoidance as the client. However, empathic listening, and help with decision-making, may go some way towards easing the distress of the husband or wife of the dementing patient.

Some relatives will value a supportive relationship, lasting throughout the course of the illness, or until a long-term arrangement has been put into effect. For others, the social worker might offer help at the time of onset, and then remain in the background, ready to liaise with other agencies or obtain concrete forms of assistance when these are requested. Referral to either a voluntary self-help organisation or a supportive small group may be appreciated. However, the focus of these may be unwelcome to some relatives, since they may be afraid that membership of such groups will have the effect of intensifying their distress and preoccupation. It is certainly important for the relatives of these younger patients to develop roles for themselves other than as devoted spouse or parent of the sufferer, but all too common for them to withdraw from social and family life, children, and attention to their own future. It is possible for the patient-centred professional to be guilty of influencing the relatives in the direction of reluctant and resentful martyrdom.

In conclusion it bears repeating that all the organic disorders can be accompanied by other symptoms – probably anxiety and depression are the most frequent. They place enormous strain on the family. Their effects are exacerbated by social stigma, and by our failure to provide the varied services which we know would help ease the situation. Because no cure can be found for the basic disorder, that is no justification for not giving help with other difficulties. The danger is, that faced with something so distressing and intractable as a major failure of mental function, the professional is made to feel powerless and is tempted to withdraw.

Mental disorder associated with epilepsy

Epileptic seizures result from pathological neuronal discharge, the causes of which are extremely varied. The seizures range from major convulsions to momentary loss of consciousness. Mental disorder occurs in only a minority of people with epilepsy. Epilepsy is a frightening illness, not only for the sufferer but also for others around him, and much anxiety and depression is readily understandable, in view of the difficulties that so many of these patients suffer over and above the epilepsy itself. Even when the seizures are well controlled by medication – and this is usually the case – the person is often cruelly stigmatised. His life-style is con-stricted: many jobs, leisure activities and modes of travel may be impossible; and restrictions are often added to unnecessarily by family or employers, as much out of ignorance as prejudice. The social worker might be involved in attempting to clarify matters for the key people in the patient's life. The patient himself might benefit from membership of a specialist self-help organisation.

It is true that in certain forms of epilepsy there is a raised risk of personality disorder of the types labelled as paranoid, explosive, or inadequate, and of psychosis closely resembling schizophrenia; but such cases are rare. Also rare are manifestations of brain damage due to epilepsy, which can take the form of intellectual impairment, emotional difficulties, or behaviour disorders, all of which may be either acute or chronic.

Although it is important for social workers to know about these possibilities, it is equally important to bear in mind the figures quoted by Anderson and Trethowan (1973): one-sixth of patients with epilepsy, treated in general practice in Britain, suffer from neurotic or stress disorders; 10 per cent need psychiatric treatment in a hospital at some time, usually only for a short period; but three-quarters of all chronic epileptic patients are fully employed. The norm, then, is for the person with epilepsy to be free of mental disorder, and to cope with his life as competently as anyone else. In assisting the individual sufferer, we must assume mental normality unless there is good evidence to the contrary; otherwise we run the risk of laying a further burden of anxiety on the person and his family.

Part 2

General Issues

10

The Children of the Psychiatric patient

The children of some psychiatric patients are at a disadvantage from the very beginning of their lives. Some are vulnerable because of genetic factors (see Tsuang and VanderMey, 1980; Gunderson *et al.*, 1974). However, there is considerable evidence that women with severe mental disorder are more likely to experience complications during pregnancy and childbirth than other mothers. Complications result from self-neglect, failure to make use of medical services, and anxiety about the birth; but the reactions of obstetricians to these mothers, such as greater use of medication, and other means of hastening delivery may be partly to blame (for a summary of research on this topic see Garmezy, 1974).

Childbirth is one of the stress experiences that can trigger a major mental illness (puerperal psychosis), especially severe depression, or rarely, schizophrenia. Much more commonly, a minor form of depression ('the blues') may follow childbirth. Even a mild form of mental disorder may cause a subtle disturbance in the manner of relating to the new-born child. Since new mothers are already under medical surveillance, they are likely to receive prompt treatment and help and support from nursing staff. Nevertheless, the foundations for later childhood disorders could be laid at this crucial period.

This chapter is about the effects of parental mental disorder at a later stage, when – all too often, it seems – the attention of professional staff may be focused exclusively on the parent.

First, a few words from the children themselves:

She is quite a nice mother, really. She doesn't do anything bad. She doesn't hit or anything. She just sits. She is like a kid mostly. When I give her a lot of candy she just sucks it up like a vacuum cleaner. She doesn't comb her hair and her dress has spots on it. Sometimes she laughs at me and I am not making any jokes. I say: 'Mom, why are you laughing at me?' and she just laughs more. I don't like it when she laughs like that. It's not like real laughing. She never used to be like that when I was little. She was just ordinary. (Anthony, 1969)

You cannot believe what it's like to wake up one morning and find your mother talking gibberish. (Anthony, 1969)

I am afraid when Mom takes a long time to come home. She tried to commit suicide because of my Dad. It wasn't until long after the divorce she stopped crying. I think of her jumping off the Golden Gate Bridge. (Wallerstein and Kelly, 1980)

Like other adults in the child's environment, social workers in adult psychiatry have often been too preoccupied with the patient to pay much attention to the child. The separation between child psychiatry and adult psychiatry is part of the problem: many adult psychiatrists do no more than ask whether there is someone to look after the children when the patient is admitted. One advantage of 'generic' social work is the possibility of offering a better service for the family as a whole. In ignoring the experiences of these children, we are forgoing the opportunity to try to help with the pain that lies close to the surface in statements like those quoted above.

Social workers need to think about the child's welfare from several perspectives. They have to assess present pain and how to alleviate it. They have also to consider the possible sequelae later in childhood and in the longer term as well. The details of an individual child's experience can be distressing in the extreme; or we can be touched and impressed by the resilience of traumatised children, and the staying power of parental love and care even when other facets of the parent's mental life are seriously disrupted.

We begin with a brief summary of some research studies showing correlations between parental mental disorder and disorder in children. It must be stressed that these are generalisations only; but they serve to alert us to situations of possible risk to children. The mechanisms whereby risk is translated into actual harm require much more detailed analysis than they have received to date. However, some pointers do emerge that can help in the assessment of individual families. The possibilities for compensating for the disadvantage of having a mentally disturbed parent have only recently begun to be explored, but the research and practice-based literature is beginning to yield some guidelines as to how present pain might be alleviated, and future difficulties reduced if not altogether prevented.

The children of the mentally disordered have a raised risk of psychological disorder, both during early and later childhood (Rutter, 1966; Rutter *et al.*, 1975; Rutter, Quinton and Yule, 1977; Richman, 1977; Rice, Ekdahl and Miller, 1971; Cooper *et al.*, 1977). For example, Cooper *et al.* (1977) found that 45 per cent of patients' children suffered from psychiatric disorder, as opposed to 26 per cent of children in the control group; figures from some other studies are even higher, but we should note that different criteria are used by different researchers. School behaviour problems, reading difficulties, and absenteeism from school have also been associated with parental psychiatric disorder (Kolvin *et al.*, 1977). Studies of child abuse and neglect have repeatedly found a greater-than-chance association with parental disturbance (Smith, Hanson and Noble, 1973; Baldwin, 1977). Studies of family burden (Hoenig and Hamilton, 1969; Grad and Sainsbury, 1968) emphasise the adverse effects upon children in the household of a psychiatric patient.

Several researchers conclude that the diagnosis or severity of the parent's disorder may be less significant than are problems of family interaction and the way a child may be 'caught up' in the parent's symptoms (see, for example, Rutter 1966), and some of these factors will be discussed later. Nevertheless, there are a number of findings concerning the different diagnostic categories that are worth noting, since they highlight possible contexts for the development of children's problems. Again, we should bear in mind that these studies provide hypotheses to be considered in the individual case, not certain predictors.

Taking 'personality disorders' first, several studies of battering parents (for example, Smith, Hanson and Noble, 1973; Baldwin, 1977) have found a very high proportion of people with this diagnosis. West and Farrington (1973) found that 'severe abnormality of personality' in a parent was strongly associated with delinquency. Among others, Rutter (1966), Wolff and Acton (1968), and Rutter, Quinton and Yule (1977) have found a strong correlation between parental 'personality disorder' and psychiatric disorder in children.

The children of alcoholics are similarly at risk, especially with regard to aggressive-conduct disorders (Stewart, DeBlois and Cummings, 1980). Wilson (1981), reviewing this literature, lists the ill effects associated with alcoholism in a parent as follows: abuse and neglect of the child, and children's problems, particularly under-achievement, developmental disorders, fearfulness and social isolation. She comments that such problems may be equally common among the children of parents with other types of disorder, but that delinquency, truancy and aggression do seem to be more common in this group. Another association, which is supported by a considerable body of evidence, is that the sons of alcoholic fathers stand a higher chance of themselves developing severe alcoholic problems when they grow up: this is true even of those who are reared apart, and there is therefore good reason to believe that there is a hereditary component at least as regards severe drinking problems (Tsuang and VanderMey, 1980).

A recent study has found a high incidence of depressive symptoms among the children of severely depressed patients (McKnew *et al.*, 1979). Weissman, Paykel and Klerman (1972) found that the parenting abilities of women with depression were adversely affected. Again, there is a raised risk of physical harm to the children of these patients. Anxiety and milder forms of depression, and other neurotic disorders in parents, have also been implicated in children's school-behaviour problems: reading difficulties, absenteeism from school (Kolvin *et al.*, 1977) and neurotic symptoms (Garmezy, 1974) The children of phobic parents often acquire fears similar to their parents (Marks, 1969; Windheuser, 1977).

Psychotic disorders in parents were less strongly implicated than neurotic and personality disorders in Rutter's (1966) study of the children of sick parents. Rutter suggests the following explanation for this finding: (a) there was a higher probability of the other parent being healthy; (b) there was less likelihood of marital discord than was the case for people with neurosis or personality disorder; (c) the patient was more often hospitalised, so that there was perhaps less strain on the family. However, more recent studies (Rice, Ekdahl and Miller, 1971; Newman, 1970; Cooper *et al.*, 1977) have noted a variety of serious problems and undoubtedly distressing experiences when children are brought up by psychotic mothers; and Garmezy (1974), in a comprehensive review of the research, concludes that the children of psychotic parents reveal a broader range of disturbance, when compared with the children of neurotic parents who show mainly a raised incidence of neurotic symptoms. Some psychotic parents are either temporarily or permanently unable to provide even basic physical care (Garmezy, 1974). A small number of psychotic parents may attack their children, usually as a result of delusional beliefs involving the child (Smith, Hanson and Noble, 1973).

In severe psychiatric disorders, and to a lesser extent other disorders as well, a major problem, both for researchers, and for social workers trying to make decisions about whether a child should remain at home, is the problem of disentangling the effects of other variables. These children may be at risk because of their genetic endowment, temporary separations from their family, or the shortcomings of temporary substitute care. The chances of developing schizophrenia, manic-depressive illness, or severe alcohol problems in later life, are little affected, whether the child remains at home or not (Tsuang and VanderMey, 1980). But being brought up by a disturbed parent does not improve the child's prospects, and can frequently lead to neurotic problems, behaviour disorder or delinquency; and we have to add to this list the blatant fact of 'present pain' caused by ill-treatment and neglect (whether deliberate or otherwise), stigma, confusion, and anxiety. And despite the large amount of literature documenting the effects of maternal deprivation, there is increasing evidence that children placed in long-term foster care, or adopted, can recover from the effects of their earlier damaging experience and achieve nearly their full potential (Clarke and Clarke, 1976).

The social worker's dilemma is often heightened by the knowledge that the parent will suffer deeply if the child is taken away. This dichotomy of interests is perhaps greater where the parent is mentally ill than in other child-care cases – the child may literally be all that parent has left to live for. The problem can be exacerbated by a division of loyalty between the various professionals, the adult psychiatrist arguing on behalf of the parent ('The loss will add to her disturbance or cause a relapse; she has suffered so many losses already'), while the child psychiatrist or the social worker emphasises the present hurt and potential damage to the child.

In assessing these situations, we may find that the clients themselves have clear-cut, reasoned views: children may wish to leave home, parents may accept that they cannot cope. More often, parents will want to keep their children, and children will want to remain, or will show a painful ambivalence. If – as is generally accepted – the 'child's best interests' are to take precedence, a detailed assessment of the child's development and his state of mind is needed. However, the presence or absence of visible signs of distress can sometimes be misleading. Tonge (quoted by Cooper *et al.*, 1977), in a study of problem families ('families in turmoil'), found that those children who showed symptoms were more likely to cope well when they grew up than children who appeared normal and well-adjusted; the latter more likely to repeat their parents' patterns. Whether this finding will be duplicated by further research, and whether it holds true for other types of 'families in turmoil', remains to be seen, but it should alert us to the necessity of considering not just the child's apparent reactions, but also the situations to which he is exposed, and especially the patterns of interaction within the family, the care he receives, and the behaviour he witnesses.

Severely disturbed behaviour

When the parent suffers from severe mental illness and behaves in a bizarre and unpredictable manner, at least a temporary separation is inevitable. Usually the parent will be admitted to hospital. In cases of hypomania, severe depression and some cases of schizophrenia, recovery can be quite rapid and the family is soon reunited. However, as short admissions become increasingly the rule even when recovery is far from complete, more and more parents, especially those with chronic schizophrenia, are living at home despite being still severely handicapped.

In the study by Creer and Wing (1974) most of the schizophrenic parents had difficulties with the care of their children, and the spouse often had to take on a large share of the parental tasks. Creer and Wing suggest that major problems arise when the spouse is not able or willing to do this. Apart from irritability and lack of supervision, the informants mentioned instances of the patient talking to the child about delusions, answering hallucinatory voices in the child's presence, and threatening suicide. A study by Newman (1970) describes a mother holding her baby upside down to feed him, and another taking her school-age child to school in a pram. Just how common such extreme situations are is difficult to estimate: they should certainly be borne in mind as possibilities. Less bizarre, but probably equally stressful, instances from the author's experience include the children of a paranoid mother who were kept locked in the house with her for days on end, and the husband with delusional jealousy who constantly cross-questioned his children about their mother's imagined infidelity.

It is important to acknowledge to the child that his parent's behaviour must be distressing and confusing. These children need to develop an understanding beyond their years of what has happened and how to interpret the parent's actions. Like many of the people around him, both grown-ups and other children, he may see 'mad' as 'bad', or may perhaps blame himself. He may adopt a facade of not caring, or of even being derisive. The younger child often accepts his parent's statements at face value. Someone who takes time to clarify the situation, to listen to his worries, and anticipate the questions he is too frightened to ask, can do a great deal to help. Above all, it is essential to demonstrate care and respect for the sick parent.

The social worker may be the only person who can undertake this role, but we should take every opportunity to help a relative – especially the other parent – to take it on, perhaps by giving the lead in a three-way discussion, perhaps by helping to rehearse the task beforehand. There is a danger of usurping the role of parent or grandparent or older sister or brother; it may be that one of these, helpless in the face of the patient's illness, will gain some comfort and sense of purpose through being able to provide help to the child. Where the child is in care outside his own family, the same considerations apply: the person involved might be a foster parent or a residential social worker.

When parent and child are apart, difficulties can arise over the question of meetings. The care-giver often needs considerable support, especially in disentangling his own feelings of resentment and alarm about mental illness from realistic concern about the effects such meetings might have on the child. Sometimes, especially with younger children, compromises are inevitable, and could call for alternative ways of preserving contact: messages delivered by another adult as go-between, letters, photographs, or visits that are very carefully monitored, and curtailed if the parent becomes disturbed. If a visit proves distressing, someone must be available to talk things over with the child afterwards.

Mental disorder can lead to stigmatisation of the whole family.

The 'odd' lady who is shunned in her village may have children who dare not go out to play. Other children in a children's home may cause much suffering to the one whose visiting parent 'talked crazy'. Apart from important long-term efforts to improve the public's (and that includes children's) understanding and tolerance, there are ways in which we might help individual children to cope. Patients in an adolescent psychiatric unit have been helped via social skills training to deal with hostility or derision from their classmates (Canever, 1980), and such assistance could be extended to some of the children of the mentally disordered.

Teenagers often become aware of the possibility of inheriting mental disorder, and can become very afraid for their own sanity or that of their future children. Genetic counselling at a specialist centre is becoming increasingly available. Tsuang and VanderMey (1980) give a helpful account of the processes by which mental disorder may be transmitted, and the risks for various disorders: schizophrenia, mania and depression, pre-senile dementias and alcoholism. They also describe the process of genetic counselling. Besides assessing the risk in the individual case, the varying 'costs' in terms of suffering and disability associated with the different disorders are explained, and the client is helped to make a personal decision about whether he would wish to avoid becoming a parent. Such advice is likely to be reassuring for most clients, and in the rare cases where the risks of inheritance are high and predictable (for example, in Huntington's Chorea families, or in the case of a person with two schizophrenic parents), the client will at least be spared the pain of inexpert and unplanned revelations.

Anthony (see account in Garmezy, 1974) has developed a programme of intervention with the children of severely disturbed parents. The procedures are classified as 'crisis' and 'precrisis' measures. Crisis measures include talking over stressful experience and the fears, guilt, confusion and ambivalence associated with the psychotic parent; and discussions of rational and realistic attitudes and behaviour. Special attention is paid to problems the child may have in sorting out reality from delusions, and in coping with both separations and reunions. Schools are involved in an all-round endeavour to anticipate the special needs of these children. The precrisis measures include opportunities of making relationships with other adults and developing skills in a wide range of activities, training of the family as a whole in problem-solving skills, and education about the nature of mental illness. Anthony's programme would seem to have much to offer, especially for those whose parent is severely disturbed.

Physical abuse and neglect

As we have noted, a small minority of psychotic parents may hurt their children during an acute phase of their illness. Others may be unable to meet their basic needs. However, child abuse and neglect are more often found in families where one or both parents are diagnosed 'personality disordered' or 'psychopathic'. (These elastic and often tautologous labels mean that varying proportions of parents are so designated according to the practice of the particular investigator.) The prospects of helping such parents to change seem remote in our present state of knowledge. Long-term 'relationship work', combined with provision of material help in order to reduce stress, is the commonest approach. Behavioural workers attempt to train the parents to manage their children more effectively, so that there are fewer situations that could trigger violence; alternatively, the parent is taught ways of dealing with stress and anger-provoking stimuli in other ways. Unfortunately, the closer the parent's behaviour approximates to that of the 'true' psychopath, the less likely it is that he will co-operate, or be able to develop control of aggressive impulses or persevere with new coping strategies. The decision as to whether children should live with these parents will be facilitated if social workers negotiate a clear behaviour-change contract and monitor its fulfilment or otherwise (Stein, Gambrill and Wiltse, 1974).

Similar problems can occur with parents who have a serious drinking problem, although at least some protection can be afforded by parents who learn to avoid their child at times when their self-control is impaired by alcohol (Wilson, 1981).

Abuse and neglect associated with depression may well cease when the depression is treated. In these cases, too, compensatory services for the child might be of value, and practical help to reduce stress on the parent, such as babysitting, nurseries, home helps and homemaker services, may act indirectly as a means of protecting the child.

Lack of stimulation

Another form of neglect that is often singled out is lack of stimulation, which is particularly detrimental to the development of younger children. Playing with the child, talking to the child, and warm physical contact may all be reduced, although the basic feeding, washing, and so on may still be carried out efficiently. Mothers who are depressed or withdrawn, or distracted by severe anxiety, may be particularly impaired in this key aspect of parenting. Whether there are critical stages in the child's life after which these lacks cannot be compensated for remains unclear, although there are indications that children who are disadvantaged at an early stage can indeed catch up with normal development later on (Clarke and Clarke, 1976). However, it may be possible to identify and try to compensate for understimulation at the time it first begins to be a problem. If another family member is not available to act as 'supplementary parent', outside help may have to be enlisted.

The burden on the child

The burden on the children is especially heavy in families where one or both parents are so disabled as to be incapable of coping with household tasks, and more important, with the care and control of the child's younger brothers and sisters. Although little has been written on the subject, it seems that this is most likely to occur in homes where a parent is disabled by chronic psychotic illness or severe alcoholism. A book written specially for the children of alcoholics, *How to Cope with an Alcoholic Parent* (Seixas, 1980), highlights the burden they carry whilst offering both practical suggestions and information about the condition.

Apart from tiredness, and missing out on activities such as playing and school-work, these children may seem contented enough, until they enter another environment. But their habitual controlling of others, and their work-orientation, can make them unpopular, and they may have considerable difficulty in 'becoming a child again'. These children often demand to be reunited with a sick parent, whom they promise to take care of. Such children need a lot of help if they are to relinquish the one role and take another that is more age-appropriate. Reassurance that the parent is all right without them will not be sufficient.

Modelling

Another worrying feature of homes where a parent is mentally disturbed is the modelling of bizarre or maladaptive behaviour. Young children sometimes repeat delusional statements, and give every indication of believing what they are saying. The content of delusions is often frightening, so that the child becomes very anxious, as well as getting himself labelled as 'crazy' by other children. With the very young, it may be necessary to talk about what is 'make believe', but even older children often need help in distinguishing the illness-related statements of the parent.

Perhaps equally damaging are the effects of anxiety in the parent, especially phobias and agoraphobia. Windheuser (1977), in a paper entitled 'Anxious Mothers as Models for Coping with Anxiety', confirms the association between anxiety in the mother and in her child, and the similarity in the objects of their anxiety. Further, he demonstrates the importance of treating the mother as well as the child. Children who received standard behavioural treatment (desensitisation with relaxation, *in vivo* exposure, verbalised self-instruction, and reinforcement for progress helped by the mother as co-therapist) showed less improvement than those whose mothers were themselves treated, modelling how to co-operate in therapy.

Although obsessional and other neurotic disorders have received less attention from researchers, it seems likely that similar findings might be obtained.

Anxiety

Parental anxiety may involve the child in other ways, besides modelling. For example, school 'refusal' may be related either to irrational anxiety about the child, or to the mother's fear of being left alone (a common feature of agoraphobia). Sometimes the child is kept away from school for such reasons, rather than because of genuine anxiety on the child's part – although that can develop later if absence from school is prolonged; the child may of course be a very willing partner in this! Alternatively, the child may be infected with the mother's anxiety about herself, and afraid of what might happen to her in his absence. Some children are kept in at other times as well: one patient with obsessional disorder refused to allow her children to play outside, in case they got dirty; she also insisted on prolonged bathing, and kept the children in their nightclothes in the evening and at weekends. If such parents cannot be successfully treated (and as we have seen, the prospects for this are improving as behavioural methods are used more widely), it may be necessary to arrange for separation.

So far in this chapter the focus has been on those situations or mechanisms that are comparatively easy to recognise. Other, more insidious, mechanisms have also been proposed as responsible for the harm suffered by children of psychiatric patients.

Marital problems

Marital problems are suggested by several investigators as a key intervening variable between mental disorder and its consequences for the child (Rutter and Hersov, 1976), though it is important to note that not all children's disorders develop in families where there is marital discord, and that marital discord does not always result in disturbance in the children (Hetherington and Martin, 1972). While there are many possible ways in which the two sets of problems might be connected, the list of 'plausible hypotheses' suggested by Hetherington and Martin provides a starting point for analysis: (a) simple displacement of anger from spouse to child; (b) antagonism between the spouses coming to centre on child care; (c) one parent trying to get the child as an ally against the other; (d) one parent reacting with helplessness and withdrawal, and encouraging the child to take on adult responsibility. Marital counselling is one possible approach to the problem, but we should not be over-optimistic, bearing in mind Crowe's (1978) finding that when one member of a couple has a psychiatric history, such treatment is less likely to be effective. Hetherington and Martin (1972) suggest that helping one or both parents to understand how their disputes affect the child might in itself be helpful. Another possibility is to try to provide a warm, consistent relationship with another adult.

Other problems of parent–child interaction

Problems of parent–child interaction need not necessarily be mediated through marital problems. Certain patterns have been identified in the homes of disturbed children, and it seems likely that these patterns are more common where a parent is mentally disordered. Patterson, Cobb and Ray (1973) give a detailed description. The 'diffusion' parent is inattentive to the antecedents in a chain of problem behaviour, eventually reacting, but inconsistently and ineffectively. Such parents fail to attend to appropriate behaviour on the child's part. Parents who are depressed, withdrawn, distracted by anxiety or generally 'inadequate' are likely to fit this picture. Patterson, Cobb and Ray comment that such parents have difficulty in following through a programme to reduce the child's problem behaviour.

The second type described by these workers is the 'selective diffusion' parent. These parents fail to deal with problem behaviour, though they do reinforce appropriate behaviour. They might be called overindulgent, and it is suggested that this pattern often has its roots in the desire to compensate the child for some real or imagined neglect or misfortune. These situations are common in families where separations or other stressful experiences have occurred due to parental mental illness. Either or both parents might develop this pattern.

The third pattern described by Patterson, Cobb and Ray is the 'sado-masochistic'. One parent takes a punitive role and the other tries to 'make up' by being warm and tolerant no matter what the child does. When the harsh parent is present, the child is punished severely; when he is absent, the child's behaviour is out of control. The mentally disordered parent might take either role: for example, the problem drinker, and the depressed or over-anxious person, might indulge the child, whereas the psychopathic or the obsessional might be especially harsh and intolerant.

Baumrind (1967) studied parent–child interaction in an attempt to analyse patterns of child care associated with children described as 'energetic–friendly', 'conflicted–irritable' and 'impulsive–aggressive'. The parents of the 'energetic–friendly' children differed from the rest in that they could resist pressure from the children, were willing to exert control and make demands, and were also willing to enter into discussion with the child; and they used more positive reinforcement and less punishment. The parents of the 'conflicted–irritable' group were less capable of exerting control, and this was combined with fewer maturity demands and less nurturance. The parents of the 'impulsive–aggressive' children were less persistent in control than either of the other groups, made fewer maturity demands, but tended to be more nurturant and to use less punishment. Although the children in this study were not themselves psychiatric patients, it has been suggested (Hetherington and Martin, 1972) that the second group, the 'conflicted–irritable' children, are 'a high risk group for severe personality disturbance at a later stage'. Although there are clearly many possible precursors of this form of child management, it seems likely that parents with depression, or indeed with any disorder leading to withdrawal and low energy, might fall into this pattern of *laissez-faire* and lack of warmth.

All of these possible mechanisms are subtle and hard to spot; they may well be impossible to alter, or even to counterbalance with the provision of alternative experience for the child. However, if we can specify the problems, we are taking a first step in the direction of providing suitable help.

Both the situations and mechanisms described earlier, and these latter, more complex ones, help to account for the prevalence of disorder in the children of the psychiatric patient, and add to the possible effects of heredity and separations. Our awareness of possible harm to the child, and how it may come about, should lead us to investigate more carefully if a patient has children. The presence of another, 'well', parent may enable us to enter a therapeutic alliance, to alleviate the child's distress and prevent disorder later on. If the patient is a single parent, or both parents are mentally disturbed, the task will be considerably harder.

11

Work and Money

Work and money, the subject of this chapter, and accommodation, discussed in the next, are topics of importance for almost all social work clients. Difficulties in finding or keeping a job, and poverty and unsatisfactory housing, usually exist quite independently of any mental disorder. However, they add to the overall handicap suffered by the psychiatric patient, and to the burden on the family; they can also contribute substantially to the onset and course of the patient's disorder. From another viewpoint, a mental disorder can itself lead to these problems, as well as being affected by them. In a survey of destitute men at a reception centre, it was estimated that 26 per cent were alcoholics, 22 per cent suffered from personality disorder, and 18 per cent suffered from mental illness. Prior to their first hospital admission, most of the mentally ill had been living in a normal domestic setting. Of those who had left hospital during the preceding year, nearly one-third had come to the centre within less than a week, another quarter within three months, and another quarter within six months (Tidmarsh and Wood, 1972). It is estimated that of a total of 60,000 schizophrenics living in the community in Britain, 5,000 are destitute (Office of Health Economics, 1979). These findings illustrate how psychiatric patients can drift down the social scale. They also demonstrate how people with disorders that have not responded to treatment may be deprived of other kinds of help as well. It is true that the destitute are a tiny minority of all those who suffer from mental disorder; but, for each of these, there are many more who have difficulty in the spheres of work, money, or housing, and who receive less help than they need.

Apart from the fact that such difficulties may worsen the chances of a lasting recovery from mental illness, there is the straightforward

moral point of view that people should not suffer a double disadvantage in comparison with the more fortunate members of our
society; and as Wing (1978) points out, 'We should not need the
argument that poverty or unemployment or bad housing cause
psychiatric disorders in order to initiate social action.'

This chapter and the next seek to highlight these three issues
selectively in relation to the mentally disordered.

Work

The vast majority of people who have received psychiatric treatment
will return to their previous job and take up where they left off.
Others will take some time to regain work skills or recover their
confidence; then they will have to seek a new job, possibly in the face
of prejudice amongst employers and, if there is a shortage of work,
the problem of competition for any job at all. For those with a
chronic or relapsing condition, it will be necessary to consider
whether a return to work is feasible, and the type of work the person
is able to cope with. For some of these, a long period of preparation
in a sheltered setting will have to precede re-entry into open employment. It is with this last-mentioned group, composed mainly of
chronic schizophrenic patients, that the greater part of the rehabilitation literature is concerned. Other groups who experience a high
rate of unemployment are people with a diagnosis of 'personality
disorder', and alcoholics (Rutter *et al.*, 1976; Royal College of
Psychiatrists, 1979).

For most people, jobs should be satisfying in many obvious ways.
But some studies are less than reassuring. For example, in the classic
study of industrial workers in the USA (Kornhauser, 1965) large
numbers of the car workers showed feelings, attitudes and behaviour
that signified 'none too satisfactory life adjustments or mental
health'. Further, their mental-health rating varied according to the
type of job, with those in low-level, repetitive work showing the
most strain and dissatisfaction. Kornhauser's analysis supports the
view that the job was affecting the person, rather than the person's
prior characteristics influencing the type of work he obtained. Of
course, such findings do not imply that being employed is more
deleterious to mental health that being unemployed. Many studies
have linked unemployment with the onset of psychiatric symptoms

in people who were previously well (see, for example, Meacher, 1971; Hill, 1978). Work is consistently cited as a major source of self-esteem and satisfaction. The mentally ill suffer as a result of being unemployed in the same way as the rest of us. Indeed its ill effects will be felt more keenly by people who are already stigmatised in our society. Conversely, they may value the opportunity to work more highly, because it demonstrates to the world that they are no longer mentally disabled. There may be arguments of a more specific nature. Brown and Harris (1978) have shown how employment outside the home can act as a protection against the onset of depression in women. The research by Vaughn and Leff (1976) suggests that spending time apart from one's family can protect against relapse in the case of schizophrenic patients in 'high expressed emotion' homes, and this may also be true of patients with depression. The work on institutionalism by Wing and Brown (1970) has clearly demonstrated the value of activity for the chronic schizophrenic patient in reducing the degree of apathy, withdrawal and poverty of speech. Others have shown that bizarre and antisocial behaviour can be lessened by engagement in activity (see Olsen, 1979a, for a review). Occupational or industrial therapy can serve these purposes, but without providing the additional benefits of self-esteem and the esteem of others that paid work can bring. Nor should we underestimate the power of the wage packet: lack of financial incentive, rather than lack of ability, may be the reason for low levels of productivity among chronic psychiatric patients (Carstairs, O'Connor and Rawnsley, 1956).

For a small minority of patients, against these potential benefits must be set a variety of potential risks. There is increased possibility of relapse at times of important life-changes, and return to work is one such. People who take a lower-status job than they held previously may experience a lasting sense of failure and humiliation. Those who do not succeed in keeping their job may suffer disappointment and shame.

Adverse conditions at work can take many forms. This is a very individual matter, just as job satisfaction is. Overstimulation is a possibility at the work-place, including the features of social interaction subsumed under the term 'high expressed emotion'; understimulation can also occur. A person may suffer from isolation if he works too much alone, or from its converse, too close contact with other people. Shift-work can disrupt family and social life. Stress can result from pressure to work fast, a noisy atmosphere, frequent demands for adaptation and change, or the behaviour of colleagues. Some jobs will be experienced as boring, or there may be too much variety. Some tasks will be felt to be demeaning.

The social worker seeking to help with a job problem has to liaise with a large number of other workers in hospital, day-centres, rehabilitation and training schemes, and employment agencies, as well as with potential employers. Some large hospitals have a comprehensive job-resettlement programme: after assessment and training on the premises, they offer a job-finding service by staff with personal contacts among local employers, and follow-up groups where ex-patients can discuss their experience and encourage one another. Social workers in areas where such facilities do not exist can learn a great deal from accounts of their methods (see, for example, Wing *et al.*, 1972; Murray, 1977).

Employment is a two-sided affair: a sensible assessment and appropriate planning require a thorough analysis not only of the wishes, attitudes and abilities of the individual, but also of the demands, potential risks and potential benefits involved in any particular job.

The individual's preferences have to be elicited, and it is necessary to talk about these in very specific terms. Exactly the same task can seem uninteresting and degrading to one person and satisfying to another, and jobs that on the surface seem to belong to the same general category can have very different meanings. Some of the meaning derives from the task, and other parts of it from the social contacts and from the status of belonging to a favoured organisation. Thus, one man who despised road-sweeping got a lot of satisfaction out of being a refuse-collector; another objected to 'domestic work', but was delighted with a caretaker post. Theatre porters in hospitals often derive much satisfaction from their helping role. Similarly, work as a shop assistant covers a wide range of possible meanings. In relation to the task itself, it is interesting to note that Remploy, the British state-sheltered workshop, offers mentally disabled workers a better chance of undertaking complex work than does open industry (Wansbrough *et al.*, 1979).

Some patients who are reluctant to return to work may be suffering from loss of confidence in their ability, rather than a genuine deficiency in work-related skills. This is a common consequence of 'being a mental patient', rather than of mental illness in itself. Social workers may be able to help by analysing the sources of this anxiety and devising a plan to help overcome it. A step-by-step return via sheltered work might be advisable, or some other anxiety-reduction programme on an individual or group basis. Apart from rehearsal of situations that worry the client, visiting the work-place, and meeting employer or colleagues in advance, might be useful strategies. Often, just talking over the probable events of the working day, and any specific anxieties, will be sufficient. This might be backed up by promising to be available for the client to telephone or visit soon after his return to work, although, of course, it is important not to imply that one is expecting him to encounter difficulties.

Apathy, bred of institutionalism and long periods of inactivity, and perhaps compounded by the effects of chronic schizophrenia, can be harder to overcome. Again, a step-by-step approach, with gradually increasing demands and a rather active style of supervision, with immediate and consistent reinforcement, is the most promising helping strategy; this is carried out in the hospital, day-centre or sheltered workshop.

The patient's family, and their attitudes, are often very influential. Freeman and Simmons (1958) have shown that poor work performance by psychotic patients is related to living with parents, and low expectations on their part. Sharing the process of assessing the patient's abilities with the relatives might help to modify their expectations in the direction of greater realism concerning his potential.

Wing (1966), studying men at an Industrial Rehabilitation Unit, stressed the necessity for a constructive attitude – and a realistic one. Some patients (and their families) find it hard to accept that their progress may have to be slow and their aspirations lowered. Professional helpers can also err in the same direction. This is one of the most complex aspects of rehabilitation, because 'a realistic attitude' is extremely hard to define. Two sources of evidence are needed: a recent evaluation of what the person is capable of doing; and a well-founded forecast of what he is capable of withstanding.

Assessment is best done in the closest possible approximation to the actual work setting (Watts, 1978). It covers both the specific instrumental skills, and the ability to concentrate and work at a suitable rate (either of which may be impaired in patients with chronic schizophrenia or depression). Of at least equal importance are such abilities as time-keeping, readiness to follow instructions, and relationships with colleagues and supervisors. Occupational therapists, and supervisors with experience in ordinary work settings are best equipped to carry out such assessment. Alternatively, there are a few schemes which provide the opportunity to try out the job while the employer remains free of obligation to pay or retain the ex-patient. (One such scheme is described below.)

The consequences of the various kinds of work-related stress may begin to show themselves even during a limited assessment period. However, it is more often the case that a prediction has to be made on the basis of the person's previous history and the nature and course of his illness. The person's history sometimes provides clues as to what should be avoided. He may have experienced difficulties in meeting new people or having to fit in with time requirements. Some patients may have relapsed upon promotion to a post involving authority or rapid decision-making; some may have succumbed to exhaustion when they moved to a job requiring physical strength or long hours of travelling. It is extremely difficult to predict what might constitute stress in an individual case, and, in the absence of such clues, I would suggest that we do not have the right to dissuade someone from seeking the kind of work that he feels will be possible and rewarding. We cannot assume, for example, that someone who has been a secretary ought to be relegated to simple assembly work after a single episode of illness, no matter how severe. Blanket recommendations about future work are a frequent subject of complaints by schizophrenic patients and their relatives.

So far, we have discussed the importance of having a detailed profile of the client as worker and of the job itself, in order to suggest a satisfactory match, and we have taken it as read that jobs are available to be selected from. We turn now to the other part of the problem, that of finding work opportunities: job-hunting, the trial-period system, and the question of discrimination.

There is some disagreement in the literature as to whether it is best for patients to find work before they are discharged. Olsen (1976a) found that of those in his sample who worked, over half had gone direct to work from hospital. By contrast, Wansbrough and Cooper (1980) found that ex-patients referred direct from hospital to open employment lasted a shorter time in employment than those introduced from any other source, and comment that 'even a spell of unemployment seemed to offer better preparation'. There is, however, considerable agreement on the shortcomings of official employment services in Britain. For example, Olsen (1976a) found that only

14 per cent of the patients in his sample who had obtained work were placed by the Disabled Resettlement Service. There does seem to be considerable scope for advocacy with such agencies on the patient's behalf.

An effective behavioural groupwork approach to job-hunting has been developed by Azrin and his colleagues (1975). The group members are helped to follow up all available leads, to write applications, and to rehearse for interviews. More recently a method of assessing both these job-finding skills, and certain key work-skills, such as interaction with supervisors and co-workers, has been devised, and this might be used to augment the training (Mathews *et al.*, 1980). A similar approach can be used with individuals, but this would mean sacrificing some of the advantages of the group: group members help each other by building up a body of knowledge about local opportunities, and by giving each other support both during and between the sessions (the 'buddy system').

For more severely handicapped clients, sheltered work (enclaves) may be available in some areas. A similar arrangement is the 'job rehearsal' system: as an ongoing programme for a group of clients, or an individual agreement with an employer. This approach is described by Wansbrough and Cooper (1980). The responsibility for the placement remains with the 'parent organisations', who prepare and support the client, and make the work contract direct with the employer. Later, if both the client and employer are satisfied, the client becomes a regular employee. Alternatively, he may then seek work with a different firm. This system does much to reassure employers, as well as giving ex-patients an opportunity to prove themselves. A variety of similar schemes, all heavily reliant on the assistance of medical staff in the firm, and especially on the hospital's industrial liaison officer (a role normally filled by a psychiatric nurse), are described by Wansbrough (1973).

Although these are probably the best alternatives we have for hard-to-place clients, we should not be over-optimistic when it comes to helping the most severely disabled among them. (Some of the success stories recorded relate to those patients who had been in hospital unnecessarily, and took place at a time of labour shortages.) A rather different group, who are also hard to place, are those who have been out of work for very long periods and who may be handicapped by 'personality disorder'.

Wansbrough (1980) gives an account of a project offering

sheltered-work experience and skilled supervision for two groups: long-term unemployed people (not psychiatric patients, but over half were judged to be suffering from 'personality disorder'), and severely disabled psychiatric patients living in the community. Of the non-patients, twenty-eight out of eighty-five were chosen for the scheme and ten of these rejected the offer of work – at least four probably did so because of anxiety, and three because of the financial disadvantage that working would entail. Of the remaining eighteen, only three succeeded in taking up work outside the scheme. Of the forty-one patients, thirteen were placed in sheltered work, and eleven assessed as ready for this without a suitable position being found for them. The data on the thirteen were as follows: mean age 34; all but one diagnosed as schizophrenic; six of above-average intelligence, five average and three borderline. Despite the considerable effort that was put into helping them, only two achieved open employment, and three more had qualified success.

Although Wansbrough emphasises the shortcomings of the scheme – lack of time for assessment and preparation, and too short a trial period – the catalogue of problems makes sobering reading. Seven patients were considered to have been adversely affected by their work experience, their reactions ranging from psychotic relapse to a mild recurrence of symptoms. Skill deficits included being unable to use the telephone, reluctance to take initiative or accept responsibility, confusion and distractability, sleeping at work, offensive eating habits, paranoid behaviour and, especially, absenteeism and lateness. Some of the stresses experienced by the patients were: being given a stream of instructions, shift-work, having to interact with fellow workers, criticism, and pressure to work fast.

The results of this experiment bear out the view expressed by Cooper (1979), that less than half of all chronically disabled patients of working age could be employed, although the thrust of his argument, based on a review of rehabilitation schemes, is toward greater optimism with regard to this patient group.

For psychiatric patients in general, an important factor, with only a tenuous connection with the actual potential of the patient, is discrimination on the part of employers. It is less likely in the case of old employees of a firm, whose difficulties are also better tolerated than those of newcomers (Wansbrough *et al.*, 1979).

A major problem with serious mental illness is the sometimes day-to-day fluctuation in the patient's mental state; and there is evidence of frequent absenteeism, inability to cope with overtime, embarrassing or 'odd' behaviour and slowness among patients with a severe psychotic illness or alcoholism. Personality disorder in particular seems to be associated with complaints about performance, absenteeism and unacceptable behaviour (Wansbrough *et al.*, 1979). It is also at least arguable that even a minor mental illness some time in the past might present a risk in a very few occupations – for example, bus driving. Unfortunately, many employers, like the general public, tend to assume that any kind of mental disorder will inevitably produce problems. In some organisations in Britain, such as the civil service, teaching, and the health service, there seems to be a tradition of discrimination against anyone who has received psychiatric treatment, and a blanket denial of work opportunities, regardless of the individual's history, or the recommendations he presents. A report from MIND (1978) describes forty cases of people who failed to obtain a job, or were dismissed, because of a history of mental disorder, and the chief reasons given were the possibility of another breakdown or of inability to withstand stress.

Unfortunately, the social worker is often barred from taking an advocacy role in such circumstances. Where advocacy is possible, arguments can be based on the client's history, and might be combined with special pleading for someone who has already suffered in other ways. Such arguments, even when they fail to benefit the individual, might help to change the employer's attitude over time. On the difficult ethical dilemma as to whether people should be advised against revealing their history, some experienced workers feel that this may indeed be the best course of action. However, apart from the risk of dismissal if the person is 'found out', there can be considerable stress in having to conceal one's past from colleagues and employers, and certain other disadvantages too. Priestley (1979) gives the example of a girl whose colleagues learned about her illness when she relapsed, and felt they would have been much more supportive had they been aware of her vulnerability. It may be possible to take a middle way. In one experiment, employers rated patients who had been trained to describe themselves either as having been 'mentally ill' or as having had 'personal problems' which they had worked on in hospital. The employers rated the 'problems' group as more likely to obtain work (Rothaus *et al.*, 1963). An ex-patient, writing about his own experience, gives the following advice: omit details of experience on the application form, and ask for an interview; during the interview give full information, express confidence in your abilities, and do not look for sympathy (Mantus, 1973).

Whether or not concealment is felt to be necessary at the present time, social workers need to join with others working towards change in society as a whole, by supporting campaigns against discrimination. Legislation against discrimination similar to that in the USA is being advocated in Britain. Meanwhile, some trades unions and civil-rights organisations may be in a position to seek redress for the victim through the law as it stands.

But we can sometimes be over-partisan and over-optimistic in our drive to get patients back into work. If he is not ready for work, this can only result in disadvantage to the person in the long run, and the employer will be probably less receptive when next approached. We also need to ask ourselves from time to time whether we should automatically consider all kinds of work to be satisfying. At a time when status depends so much on having a paid job, and we define people largely by their job title, the question being asked is whether sharing responsibility for what happens in our society, having a framework for our daily lives, and feeling 'needed', is what really matters. It may be that for some of our clients these things might come from different sources: from playing a key role in organisations, working together with others, being necessary to other people or even to animals, plants or places. For the chronic patient, and the patient who relapses frequently, there often grows up a kind of miniature culture around a helping agency, and this is heavily influenced by the attitudes of its staff. It may be that we are making an idol of work; perhaps we should consider ways of developing an equally reasonable and, possibly, more humane set of norms and values.

Money

In previous chapters we mentioned the financial difficulties that may arise for people with drinking problems, and for those who have suffered a hypomanic episode. But 'careless spending' is only rarely the cause of financial difficulties. More often the cause is unemployment; failure to obtain welfare benefits; the exceedingly low levels of state benefits; or if the patient is employed, low wages amounting to exploitation.

Financial difficulties constitute one of the most common sources of stress for psychiatric patients and their families. Yet the problem is often overlooked by mental-health professionals. Of the relatives interviewed by Creer and Wing (1974), one-third mentioned money worries, despite the fact that this sample contained a high proportion of middle-class people and families living in an area with better-than-average services. A report by a relatives' group stresses the varied causes for concern: besides low levels of state benefit and failure to claim, they mention the 'pocket money' earnings in sheltered workshops, prescription charges, and the cost of fares to visit patients and doctors (Lloyd, 1971).

The system of state benefits makes no distinction between those who suffer from psychiatric disorder and other sick people. This is as it should be; however, in some cases it may be disadvantageous to the psychiatric patient and his family.

It is clear that many psychiatric patients do not receive the amount to which they are legally entitled. Some of the reasons for this are the same as the reasons why other entitled persons fail to claim: uncertainty about one's rights, anxiety about officialdom, apathy; but these factors are generally more prevalent among people handicapped by mental illness, especially those who have become 'institutionalised', and those who are severely ill. Difficulties can begin at the time of onset or relapse. They can often continue throughout a hospital stay. (MIND (1979) has published a useful handbook entitled *Your Money in Hospital*.) But it is the chronically disabled person in the community who is most disadvantaged. Some problems are directly connected with mental illness. For example, some ex-patients are of no fixed abode. A change of residence can result in cessation or interruption of their financial benefit. Even more serious in its consequences is a particular problem associated with psychotic illness: the person does not see himself as sick or handicapped in any way. He therefore refuses to be classified as 'sick', and insists on taking jobs that he cannot manage; he may fail to turn up to work, he may develop delusions about his workmates, or be unable to concentrate; he may be sacked, or may give up the job voluntarily. He can then be treated like anyone else who is 'voluntarily unemployed', and his benefit may be reduced. Other patients simply refuse to claim; some lose their benefit cheques; and a few spend their money immediately and unwisely. It is often extremely difficult for relatives to persuade the local benefits office to allow them to take over responsibility (National Schizophrenia Fellowship, 1974b). Some relatives do succeed, but one can only guess at the hardship experienced by the many patients who lack a helpful, resourceful and persistent family. At best, it is likely that they miss out on a number of possible 'extras', such as grants for clothes, bedding, and the like, after a long hospital stay, and grants for heating when they remain at home all day; at worst, they may be grossly underpaid, and dependent on their relatives for support.

The complexity of the system, and the particular handicaps of some of the more severely ill, make it essential that social workers pay particular attention to the receipt of benefits, and undertake liaison with social security officers. The National Schizophrenia Fellowship (1974b) has suggested the appointment of special welfare rights officers within social security agencies to take major responsibility for the financial problems of the mentally ill, or of resettlement officers in social services departments who would be notified of all discharges of long-stay patients. (The latter would concern themselves with work and housing as well as financial matters.) The Disability Alliance (Hughes, 1978) recommends special financial provision for patients discharged after a long stay in a psychiatric hospital, in the form of a resettlement grant and a resettlement allowance. Besides persistent efforts to bring the facts about poverty in general to the attention of the public and the law-makers, we need to emphasise the particular disadvantages and needs of psychiatric patients.

Meanwhile, the social worker has the responsibility to try to make the system work. This means studying the regulations with care, checking constantly, and developing a close working relationship with the social security officer. Unless this officer has special knowledge and experience of mental illness, it may be necessary to offer him both reassurance and information. It may be helpful to accompany him on visits and to be ready to act as 'interpreter' – some patients can appear deliberately unco-operative or untruthful to an officer who is trying to establish the facts of their case.

Another way of helping patients to obtain their benefit is to offer them teaching about the system, perhaps in a 'discharge preparation group'. Equally important is to provide systematic training in the relevant 'claiming behaviours', such as form-filling and asking for advice, and being appropriately assertive when they seem to be receiving less help than they should. As regards handling money, there are a small number of long-stay patients who need much more basic training: in shopping, paying bills, buying bus tickets and so on.

Those who are successful in finding and keeping a job may nevertheless continue to be poor (Olsen, 1976a). Sometimes, indeed, like other low-paid workers, especially those with heavy family responsibilities, they may be worse off than if they had remained unemployed; and the decision to take work can be an extremely difficult one. Low earnings may in part be due to reduced work capacity, and in such cases, state and voluntary schemes for compensating employers in exchange for taking on the severely handicapped worker are probably the best solution. However, it seems from some research (Olsen, 1976a) that ex-psychiatric patients, who have little bargaining power, may be used as a source of cheap labour, particularly when they take on 'unofficial' employment. Here again, only persistent advocacy and intensive help might solve the problem for an individual client; in the long run, the solution will only be found in improvements in legislation, or in special programmes developed by voluntary or statutory agencies.

Unless more can be done to assist with financial problems, hardship among patients and their families will be greater than it need be; social isolation, and lack of activity and stimulation, will be exacerbated by lack of funds for the ordinary pleasures and amenities of community living; and patients with chronic disorders will be increasingly at risk of severe poverty and homelessness. Furthermore, poverty, or the prospect of poverty, with its associated risks of housing and legal problems, can constitute a severe stress able to provoke another episode of mental illness, so that the patient continues in the vicious spiral of breakdown and downward drift.

12

Accommodation

Effects of housing on mental illness

'Could you get me somewhere better to live?' is the main symptom of what has been cynically designated 'The X-town Syndrome' (for X read the name of any area where there is widespread dissatisfaction with housing provision). When asked to assist a client to jump the housing queue one may find oneself in a moral dilemma. What evidence do we have that housing conditions can affect mental health? What sort of a case can be put forward in support of this particular client obtaining different accommodation?

First of all, we can argue that a person who has problems in coping in general ought to be spared the extra stress of poor living conditions. Beyond this, and despite the fact that much is written on this subject – and we tend to respond intuitively to the suggestion that a new place to live would make all the difference – the evidence is surprisingly thin (Wing, 1978). Because housing disadvantage is almost always associated with many other forms of disadvantage, it is difficult for researchers to separate out its contribution to illness. We sometimes have to look beyond the dwelling itself, to the person's perception of the place, and how it is experienced.

The Brown and Harris study (1978) has shown that major long-term difficulties can play a causal role in the development of depression in women. One such difficulty singled out by these researchers is that of housing: state of repair, size, location, and neighbours. Major 'life events' have been linked with the onset, or relapse, of depression and schizophrenia (Brown and Birley, 1970; Paykel, 1978; Brown and Harris, 1978). Moving house, or being disappointed in one's hopes of moving, may be such an event.

A variety of features have been studied in relation to their possible effect on mental health. Overcrowding is of particular interest, and has been linked with mental disorder (Galle *et al.*, 1972; Gove *et al.*, 1978), and with a number of other personal problems that might themselves constitute stress. It seems likely that lack of personal space is not necessarily crucial in itself, but often interacts with other problems (Freeman, 1978). For example, it can exacerbate tense relationships (Rutter and Madge, 1976). For schizophrenic patients, lack of privacy could have serious consequences: the work on 'high expressed emotion' suggests that it may be important for the patient to be able to withdraw from interaction with his family.

Conversely, social contact is also important, and can be affected for good or ill by the location and design of housing. Freeman (1978) suggests that isolation exacerbates fear and suspiciousness; and the findings of Brown and Harris (1978), concerning the value of a close, confiding relationship with husband or boy-friend in protecting against depression, suggest by extension that living near a close friend or relative might be beneficial. However, a study of three new housing estates of differing designs (Wing, 1974) concluded that there were differences in satisfaction on several measures: more 'sense of belonging to the home' in the block of flats (which had the best internal quality), more 'sense of belonging to the neighbourhood' and less sense of isolation in the squares – but there were no measurable differences in mental health among the residents. It has been proposed that dissatisfaction with neighbours is more often an accompaniment of mental disorder than a cause (Freeman, 1978).

Living in a flat, as opposed to a house, is more likely to be associated with depression in women with pre-school children, especially if it is a high-rise flat (Richman, 1977), but a more general association is as yet unproven (see, for example, Moore, 1974). One major study has tested the hypothesis that moving to a new housing estate leads to a raised risk of neurotic disorder: the hypothesis was not confirmed (Hare and Shaw, 1965). Another long-held view was that schizophrenia was caused, or partly caused, by living in poor-quality high-density housing in the inner city; but this has been conclusively refuted: it appears that the high incidence of schizophrenia in these areas is the result of 'downward drift', which shows itself in housing as it does in occupation (Dunham, 1965).

Other housing features need to be investigated further, and considerable doubt remains about their possible contribution to psychiatric disorder. For example, high levels of noise (in this case, living near an airport) have not been shown to contribute significantly (Gattoni and Tarnopolsky, 1973). To sum up: considering the evidence we have at present, it seems that housing conditions may account for only a small part of the variance in mental illness, certainly at the severe end of the continuum. Taylor and Chave (1964), quoted by Wing (1978), seem to express the opinion of most researchers and reviewers:

> Dissatisfaction with the environment might be a cause of neurotic reaction. But it is more likely to be a symptom, since a remarkably constant minority of people show both a measure of dissatisfaction and nervous symptoms, wherever they happen to live.

A few pointers emerge concerning depression and schizophrenia, but by and large the social worker who is considering whether to act as advocate for someone who wants to change his accommodation has to rely on exactly the same arguments as when working with someone who is not designated mentally ill.

Most important, perhaps, is to try to understand the individual's experience of his situation. But when there are no obvious arguments for moving, we may have to reconsider the stance adopted by social workers who have reacted against traditional psychodynamic practice, taken heed of the client's views as expressed in *The Client Speaks* (Mayer and Timms, 1970), and committed themselves to taking the client's 'presenting problem' as the problem to work on. This is unpalatable, it is arguably impracticable – but perhaps, after all, we do sometimes have to probe for an 'underlying problem'. But we must first listen carefully, then say frankly why we cannot help over housing, and then explain our reasons for asking more questions about other matters.

Placement

People who have no home, who cannot manage or are no longer welcome in their previous home, and those who need further treatment in a residential setting, are frequently referred to social workers for 'placement'. The social worker may be under considerable pressure to play his expected part in 'clearing beds' for the consultant psychiatrist. Doctors who complain about social workers' apparent unhelpfulness often fail to appreciate that this is as much due to shortage of suitable places as to any lack of concern. It is very painful for a social worker to have to send someone to a doss-house because there is nowhere else, and when implementing a policy of community care becomes a matter of mere disposal. In such circumstances, the notion of skilled assessment and selection of a suitable placement seems something of a farce. This said, the sort of analysis discussed in the chapter on employment still ought to be done: consideration of the client's wishes, needs and capacities, and the demands and advantages of the particular living arrangement. If a satisfactory match between client and placement is not possible, then, while making do with second- or third-best, we can gather information on needs and numbers, for use in a longer-term endeavour to seek out or create new resources.

A first step is to discover what the client himself considers would be most suitable. Clients 'of no fixed abode' are often thoroughly familiar with a variety of facilities, and may have strong preferences. Clients may be interested in such diverse features of accommodation as single rooms, a homely rather than a clinical atmosphere, town or country location. Accessibility to work or day-centre, and to relatives and friends, could be important. Involving the client in the placement decision can have far-reaching effects: Segal and Aviram (1978) found that this factor, independently of other variables, had a significant influence on whether sheltered-care residents were able to take advantage of opportunities to participate in the life of the outside community.

In order to assess the person's needs we have to estimate his level of coping with independent living. It cannot be assumed that this will necessarily parallel his ability to cope with the demands of employment. Some psychiatric patients do ordinary jobs while still needing a highly supervised home base, sometimes even a hospital ward; others (and this is more often the case) can run a household successfully, while remaining quite unable to go out to work. The kind of question we need to answer is, whether the person's housekeeping skills are sufficient for him to feed himself on the money he gets, keep his home reasonably clean, do the shopping and the laundry and other day-to-day tasks. This part of assessment is perhaps best carried out by an occupational therapist. Self-care skills, such as washing and dressing, the social skills needed to cope with neighbours, landlords and shopkeepers, ability to use public transport and the telephone, are also part of this picture. For some clients, being able to take responsibility for medication is particularly important, and some need oversight, so that prompt medical help can be obtained if their illness shows signs of recurring or worsening. Some estimate of the person's vulnerability to isolation will also be necessary: it could be dangerous to suppose that a person prone to depression, who has no occupation and few friends, will be better situated in a bed-sitter than a hostel. Finally, there is the question of lethargy: does this patient need to be encouraged to do things – left to himself, is he likely to spend his time doing nothing?

Of the patients referred for placement, a few will qualify on all these criteria, especially those who have recently come from an ordinary domestic setting and have recovered completely from their illness. Most of these, and certain long-stay patients who have responded to intensive help within the hospital, may only require information about housing agencies and advocacy. If they cannot compete in the housing market because of age, or inability to get work, they may need special help to obtain a room or flat through a group home or housing-association scheme.

Sheltered-care facilities

In theory, if not in practice, it is relatively easy to place people who need a permanent home because of infirmity. Homes for the elderly, nursing homes, or family fostering will be suitable, since their needs do not differ from those of similar groups who have not been psychiatric patients. Nevertheless, a great deal of diplomacy may be necessary, in order to overcome unwillingness to accept them because of their psychiatric history.

The physically frail elderly who are also suffering from dementia, and the small group of younger patients with organic disorders, who are sometimes also physically disabled, may be found a place in an old people's home or a nursing home. It is particularly important to avoid the all-too-common situation in which the staff are prone to infantilising their residents: it can happen that a person who can feed himself when he enters the home is soon behaving like a baby bird, and a similar decline occurs in other life skills. Safety versus independence (which implies risk-taking) is a big enough dilemma without having to take on board the possibility of anti-therapeutic practices in residential establishments.

Clients whose mental condition has changed little, can present particularly difficult problems if they are used to an unsettled way of life, and are unwilling or unable to take advantage of a treatment programme. These are the clients who have perhaps been admitted from a doss-house, or have been sleeping rough, and may have had a relatively short stay in hospital, if indeed they were admitted at all. The main diagnostic categories are alcoholism, and personality disorder. It seems that the best solution for them is a comfortable and accepting environment, where they will have proper food and access to medical services, and where they can form a relationship with staff at their own speed, and perhaps one day find their way back into a treatment and rehabilitation process. Such provision is hard to come by. More often, these people are discharged to a situation which will itself contribute to a further deterioration in their mental and physical health.

Clients with a drinking problem, who have 'dried out', are obviously at risk if they return to their former surroundings. They need considerable support during the first months of abstinence, and are probably best served by specialist hostels for recovered alcoholics, which provide a home, companionship and encouragement. Many of them prefer this solution to committing themselves to intensive residential treatment, and in any case might not be accepted into such a programme.

The largest group requiring placement, and about whom most has been written, are people with chronic schizophrenia, and a few with severe chronic neurosis, personality disorder, or organic disorder, who have derived all the benefit they can from hospital treatment and now require a comfortable, tolerant long-stay home, which also makes the most of their remaining capacities. Long-stay hostels, boarding-out and substitute family care, and certain group homes, all accommodate such patients, and despite the differences between these various settings, all vary along the same dimensions. Basically, there is a balance to be struck between the necessary amount of care and control, and the encouragement of autonomy.

Hostels have been characterised according to the degree to which they regulate the lives of their residents (Apte, 1968; Ryan and Hewett, 1976). Although one would like ideally to see the degree of regulation geared to the needs of each individual resident, this is difficult to achieve in a group-living situation. Each hostel has its own blend of care, oversight, stimulation and encouragement, and its preferred solution to the support-versus-control dilemma. Hewett (1979) describes the continuum, from the very restrictive regime, to the setting not unlike a family home, where the few rules are necessary for everyone's benefit. While it is true that the highly structured regime can resemble the worst type of institution, there are many patients for whom a morning call, supervision of personal care and medication, and a certain amount of chivvying, are essential, in order to support their coping efforts and to guard against increasing handicap, becoming unacceptable in the community, or relapse.

Olsen (1976b), and Segal and Aviram (1978), have shown that it is possible to provide a helpful and comfortable environment for the long-term resident outside the more expensive, purpose-built, professionally staffed hostel sector. They stress that professional support is essential, including a guarantee that the psychiatric services will intervene promptly if difficulties arise. The dangers already mentioned, of not making the most of the resident's potential, and creating a miniature anti-therapeutic institution in the community, are clearly present. Even group homes, which look like ordinary households and have no resident staff, can contain people who sit around doing nothing all day, exercise little choice or control over their own lives, take their outings as a group, and have no social contacts outside. Nevertheless, many of these establishments do provide the right blend of autonomy and support. The untrained but interested landlady or boarding-house keeper often shows concern and persistence with even the most difficult clients, and the group-home residents help each other, and are supervised and encouraged by their visiting nurse or social worker.

Hostels, boarding-out arrangements and group homes are also used as a transitional rather than a permanent placement. Even in the absence of a formal change (as opposed to 'maintenance') programme, they can foster progress towards a greater degree of independence, by gradually increasing their demands and reducing the amount of control and practical help, so that the resident can redevelop his abilities and his confidence. However, many establishments fail in their stated aim of preparing their residents for ordinary life in the community. Segal and Aviram (1978) found that despite a number of treatment programmes arranged for the sheltered-care residents they studied, only about 15–20 per cent were able to return to independent living. Undoubtedly, part of the problem is that this aim may be unrealistic in the first place: the client has already reached the limits of his potential, and cannot be expected to go further. Another reason, however, is failure to provide continuing active rehabilitation. Ryan and Wing (1979) report that in only about a quarter of the cases where it seemed desirable to try to reduce maladaptive behaviour did the hostel staff attempt to bring about change; and yet few of the residents were attending day-centres, so that there was very little being done to improve their functioning, except for medication and out-patient contacts. Pritlove (1976), studying a group home, concluded that the residents' level of functioning was maintained, but they were not progressing towards increased independence.

Residential treatment facilities

While it is impossible to draw a clear line separating 'treatment' settings from those providing just bed-and-board, companionship and supervision, there are certain establishments that have definite treatment methods. They can be described under two headings: the therapeutic community, and the behavioural (or 'token economy') regime. Neither is common in a 'pure' form, but many establishments offer a diluted version of one or the other approach, or sometimes a combination. Both differ from the conventional hospital ward, in that the regime is itself the treatment in an important sense (Millard, 1981a). Both types of regime have the potential for harm, as well as for good, possibly placing too much stress on their clients, failing to individualise them, and sometimes adopting a destructive anti-medication ideology. Both can become very inward-looking, creating a world of their own without a serious effort to promote transition to ordinary life in the community outside.

In the therapeutic community the aim is to use every situation of everyday living, but especially interaction with other people, in an attempt to help people change, mainly through developing awareness of their own behaviour and feelings and how they affect others.

The therapeutic community is permissive in many respects: bed-times, meal arrangements and so on are left for individuals to decide, and staff members' and residents' roles are deliberately blur-red, so that even major administrative decisions are taken by the community as a whole. This allows the residents to bring their habitual patterns of thinking and behaviour to a broad range of situations, and to try out new patterns. Community and small group meetings are compulsory, however, and these provide the oppor-tunity for members to receive feedback and develop insight. A wide range of group methods may be employed: there are hard-hitting, confrontation-style groups, or supportive ones, and diverse and sometimes composite treatment approaches/ideologies, ranging through group analytic, transactional analysis, bio-energetics, and 'encounter'.

Staff in therapeutic communities tend to be highly committed to their approach, and residents who stay the course become very attached to the establishment; there can be no doubt of their success in developing a community identity. Evidence about effectiveness on other measures, however, is harder to come by, largely because this type of treatment is extremely difficult to evaluate. Whiteley's (1970) study of residents with personality disorders suggests a modest suc-cess rate, associated with a more 'neurotic' than 'personality dis-order' picture, marriage, above-average intelligence and middle-class background. Those with a history of convictions, truancy and broken homes were less likely to benefit, and Whiteley suggests that being treated together with the more fortunate group members might actually be harmful. Millard (1981b) concludes that there are indications that a therapeutic community is helpful for people with neurotic disorders, personality disorders, and addictions; and Blake and Millard (1979), describing a therapeutic community in a day-centre for a more mixed group of ex-patients, have reported results that are a great deal better than their previous histories would have led one to expect.

The behavioural approach seems more suited to the chronically handicapped patients, who may be suffering from the combined effects of institutionalism and the negative symptoms of schizo-phrenia – people who are not helped and may even be harmed by insight-giving, confrontation, or close, intense interaction with other people. The treatment procedures are derived from operant-conditioning theory. Adaptive behaviours, such as self-care or social interaction, are increased by providing immediate and consistent rewards, while maladaptive behaviours, such as delusional talk, are consistently ignored. The rewards often take the form of tokens, which the person can exchange for a variety of 'back-up reinforcers'. The 'token economy' proper is much more common in hospitals than it is in the community. There are numerous controlled studies testifying to its effectiveness in bringing about change in severely handicapped, institutionalised patients, although it is not yet clear what proportion of the patients respond to these procedures, or whether the successes that have been reported are maintained in the longer term and outside the original setting (Fernandez, 1982). Henderson and Scoles (1970) have shown that psychotic men in a 'token economy' hostel can achieve considerable progress. Fairweather *et al.* (1969), whose approach is somewhat similar but not 'behavioural' in the strict sense, gives an impressive account of a graduated programme for long-stay, very handicapped patients, which included systematic training in decision-making, and carefully planned group support; the patients were eventually able to move into a house together, and run their own business.

This brief account of different kinds of placement offers some indication of what might be suitable for the individual client, although we have to accept that choice is severely limited. The need for a place to live is often, but not always, accompanied by a need for rehabilitation or continuing treatment.

The number of places for long-stay residents is very limited, and it has been suggested that one way of dealing with the problem would be to persuade some of the short-stay facilities to lower their expectations. Alternatively, more long-stay accommodation could be obtained by boarding-out arrangements (Olsen, 1976b; Smith, 1979; Segal and Aviram, 1978; Anstee, 1978), by setting up group homes (MIND, 1975; Wilder, 1978; Ryan, 1979), or housing associations (Barter, 1979). Social workers have often played a central role in obtaining a supply of accommodation, as well as in matching residents and facilities. Smith (1979) and Slater (1979) discuss the tasks involved, which go far beyond liaison and administration, and encompass assessment of the homes and the people who run them, continuous monitoring and support, complex financial arrangements which often involve more than one source of funding, and the imaginative deployment of the services of volunteers. The success achieved in settling large numbers of ex-patients in the community, especially those who have grown old in hospital, is truly impressive. For example, Smith (1979) reports that of 130 long-stay patients discharged to supported lodgings and nursing homes in a scheme organised from a small psychiatric hospital, only ten (8 per cent) had required readmission over a period of five years. Slater (1979), reviewing a similar scheme, also reports a readmission rate of 8 per cent over a fifteen-year period. Both authors stress the importance of careful selection of accommodation, and of close working relationships between all the people involved, with the social worker (hospital-based) responsible for most of the planning and liaison.

Some hostels could become more treatment-oriented with the provision of extra training for their staff (see DeRisi, Myron and Goding, 1976). The social worker might act in a teaching or consultant role, although this may also be filled by a nurse, psychiatrist, or psychologist.

Before looking for a residential placement, we ought to check local resources to see whether there might be some other way of achieving what the client requires. Day-centres can provide a regular meal, supervision, companionship, occupation, and treatment and rehabilitation services, and enable patients to continue living with their families or in other ordinary accommodation. Some combination of day care, social clubs, visits by a social worker, nurse or volunteer, and out-patient treatment, might serve the patient's needs. Even a fairly intensive treatment programme may be available without the associated housing provision: for example, it is possible to receive therapeutic community treatment in a day-centre (Blake and Millard, 1979), and behavioural treatment in a day-hospital (Liberman and Bryan, 1977).

The creation of facilities such as these, plus more volunteer help, more weekend services, and better transport provision, could ease the burden on the inadequate network of residential facilities.

Plans are under way to set up a 'campus community', where a variety of accommodation, from hospital to unsupervised flats and workshops of various kinds, will be available on the same site (National Schizophrenia Fellowship, 1979). This will make it possible to arrange a smooth transition from the most dependent situation to the least dependent that the individual is capable of achieving, with continuous monitoring along the way, and the possibility of moving backwards as well as forwards with the minimum of disruption. This solution is being advocated because of the gaps and the lack of co-ordination in the present jumble of provisions; perhaps it will provide a model of comprehensive, planned services for accommodation and employment that can be emulated elsewhere.

13

Psychiatric Emergencies, Hospital Admission and Crisis Intervention

A psychiatric emergency is defined when someone's distress or alarming behaviour, caused by mental disorder, is considered by the person himself, or by other people, to require urgent psychiatric intervention. It does not necessarily entail admission to hospital, although this is often requested.

One patient, having recovered from an episode of hypomania, discharged herself against medical advice; the social worker arrived at her home within half an hour to find her making preparations for suicide. A patient with chronic schizophrenia became incoherent and deluded, and attacked his sister. An elderly lady was found wandering at night talking in a disjointed incomprehensible fashion. All these were psychiatric emergencies defined by people other than the patient. The case of a woman who rang the hospital saying she was trembling all over and thought she was going to die, and the man who lay in bed refusing to eat and weeping quietly and asking for his doctor, also constitute psychiatric emergencies, recognised as such by the patients themselves.

In everyday language, 'crisis' means 'a turning point', but it has taken on the sense of 'emergency' as well. In the technical language of crisis intervention theory it means an event which makes excessive demands on a person's coping capacity, along with his reaction to the event. All psychiatric emergencies can fit the definition of crisis, but not every crisis is a true psychiatric emergency. To illustrate. A patient's husband discovered that his wife had been having an affair; he gave her half an hour to get out of the house. A married couple had learned that the husband had a serious progressive illness and would have to give up work; they were unable to sleep for worry. A family were in turmoil after the teenage son had been charged with breaking and entering. Although in all these cases a psychiatric patient was involved, their reaction could not be described as 'mental illness'. Nevertheless, members of the psychiatric team might wish to intervene in order to try to ease distress and prevent a further deterioration in the situation, especially if the patient is vulnerable to relapse when under stress.

In this chapter we consider first the psychiatric emergency and some key issues regarding the need for hospital admission. The second part deals with the broader topic of crisis intervention, its value and limitations in relation to psychiatric patients.

The psychiatric emergency

When the prospective patient is said to be acutely disturbed or possibly violent, most social workers will feel anxious as they prepare for the interview. If there is any likelihood of being involved in a possible compulsory admission it is essential to be prepared with the necessary legal documents. If there is a possibility of violence, it is sensible to ensure that there will be someone else present. It is of the greatest importance to allow time. Most people will calm down in due course; and time is needed for everyone to have their say, for unhurried decisions to be made, and for professional helpers to explain what is happening to the patient and the family. Even the patient who seems totally out of contact with reality may later recall everything in vivid detail; on the other hand, not only the patient but also his distraught relatives may have difficulty in taking in what is said to them at this time.

The psychiatric emergency is a situation which makes demands on a wide range of the knowledge and skills in the social worker's repertoire: his ability to interview under difficult conditions, his skill in assessing problems and needs, his legal knowledge, and his familiarity with resources in the community.

Assessment

The first task, usually shared with the doctor, is to gain a clear picture of what the emergency is about: what is it that people fear will happen unless immediate assistance is provided? How is the client feeling, what is he doing? What explanations for this can be given?

Although the judgement as to whether someone is suffering from a mental disorder is essentially a medical one, the social worker cannot avoid making a provisional judgement about this as well. As we discussed earlier (p. 10), the social worker with specialist psychiatric knowledge and experience can be extremely skilled at this screening task.

Any form of mental disorder can present a psychiatric emergency, but the most commonly met are acute schizophrenia, hypomania, severe depression, acute anxiety states (panic attacks), and disrupted or bizarre behaviour associated with organic disorder. Sometimes very disturbed behaviour is due to intoxication, which will, of course, subside quickly in most cases. If the patient is willing to accept medication, the doctor may be able to alleviate the severity of disturbance temporarily in the other conditions, although only in the case of the acute anxiety state can the patient be expected to return to normal without further treatment.

Such conditions as these have to be differentiated from severe distress (perhaps fitting the lay description 'hysterics'), anger, or deliberate social withdrawal. The so-called patient may be reacting to a family row, distressing news, or a problem which he does not wish to divulge to his relatives.

Another, particularly hard-to-handle, type of emergency is what might be called 'the manipulative crisis'. This involves threats to injure oneself (or very occasionally someone else) unless the professionals provide some service – usually a hospital bed, but sometimes help of some other kind: financial, perhaps, or housing. This type of behaviour often draws the label 'personality disorder', 'psychopathic' or 'hysterical'. It is a matter for fine judgement whether these situations constitute grounds for psychiatric intervention, and whether they ought to be treated as emergencies, crises or neither. Scott (1978) discusses such situations in a paper on kidnapping and hostage-taking. The doctor or social services department is the primary victim, and the person making the threats is both the terrorist and the secondary victim. He says 'Look after me or I shall kill myself and then you will be sorry.' Scott recommends that the negotiator does everything possible to put himself across as fair and dependable, and to avoid needlessly frustrating the person. When the person is genuinely at risk, the negotiator will consider making whatever concessions are within his power; when this is not thought to be the case, intervention (or non-intervention) can be planned, with a view to long-term, rather than temporary, solutions. We should note that often these 'contrived crises' result from someone's genuine need for help that has been previously overlooked: the relapsing schizophrenic patient who broke into a relative's house in the early hours of the morning, the mother who genuinely believed that she might harm her children and felt she must be protected against her own impulses.

Hospital admission

If psychiatric disorder is diagnosed, the next question concerns the advisability of hospital admission. The decision will depend on the gravity of the patient's condition, and the advantages of hospital observation, care and treatment in this particular case. Patients who are thought likely to endanger themselves or others (discussed in detail later in the section on compulsory admission), those who are under stress and need a respite from the demands of their home situation, and those for whom the appropriate treatment is hard to provide on an out-patient basis, are the groups most likely to be admitted to hospital. However, many other factors play a decisive role: the views of the patient and his family, the availability of beds, and the resources for community-based care, control, observation and treatment.

Whereas the doctor is best placed to assess the advantages of hospital, the social worker can contribute to the decision by considering other kinds of resource: day care, voluntary help, oversight from social services staff. In a few places, there may be alternative residential facilities which could accept the person who needs to leave his home. The social worker will also assess the family's willingness and competence to cope with the person at home – still the most used of all community resources, and perhaps the least appreciated.

Thus, the decision to admit does not depend upon a medical assessment alone. (This is true of course for physical and well as mental illness, and it is no argument against hospital admission to point this out: rather it is an argument for the community to provide more appropriate alternatives.)

A study of admissions to a London mental hospital sheds some light on present psychiatric practice (Gleisner, Hewett and Mann, 1972). A research team assessed the need for admission in a 'high risk of admission' group, and compared their judgement with what actually occurred. The main factors distinguishing those admitted were: previous compulsory admission; psychosis; severe behavioural disturbance reported by relative or patient; but not demographic factors, previous admission, or social performance. They noted that there was an interaction between behaviour and diagnosis: suicidal threats were taken more seriously in patients judged to be depressed, than in those with personality disorder. Pressure from relatives or from other professionals, availability of beds, and lack of alternative forms of care, also played an important part. The research team considered that twelve of the fifty patients who were admitted need not have been. However, several of these would have required immediate day-hospital care or a hostel place, and these alternatives were not available; others might have benefited from a crisis intervention service. Examples of these 'unnecessary admissions' included a mildly depressed mother complaining of difficulty in coping at home; a man with a serious housing problem; a single woman who felt isolated and wanted to move into a hostel; a woman with acute panic attacks who had a handicapped child and severe financial difficulties; a wife who had taken a small overdose after a marital row. This study illustrates how broad a range of problems may be felt to constitute grounds for hospital admission. An earlier study in the USA (Mishler and Waxler, 1963) found that the source of the referral, the status of the doctor making the decision, the time of day, and the number of previous admissions, all had a considerable influence.

If the patient accepts the offer of a stay in hospital, it remains for the social worker to reassure the family, and, if necessary, to make arrangements for the care of children or other dependants. Assistance may also be required with a variety of practical matters, such as payment of bills, care of pets, informing relatives, and so on.

If, however, the patient is ambivalent about going to hospital, the social worker may consider it appropriate to assist the doctor in attempting to encourage him to do so. It may be that he is afraid of what awaits him there, and the social worker who is familiar with the hospital and its staff may be in a position to offer reassurance, after getting him to say what it is he fears. When this can be done honestly, it might be helpful to point out that the time the patient is likely to spend in hospital may be quite short, perhaps reminding him of a previous occasion. Further reassurance can be given by such apparently simple measures as helping to pack a suitcase, the promise of visits, an offer to accompany him to the ward, and reassurance about the welfare of his family or the care of his property while he is away.

Sometimes a patient will refuse to go to hospital, but at the same time may show signs of wanting to accept were it not for the difficulty of 'climbing down' once having taken up a position. With tact and skill it may be possible to make room for a change of mind without humiliation.

However if the person adamantly refuses to accept admission, and there is no prospect of finding a reasonable alternative solution, then the question of compulsory admission has to be considered.

Compulsory admission to hospital

Under current English law, a social worker may have a duty to apply for admission, acting as a stand-in for the relative. He may choose to interpret his role as requiring him to safeguard the patient from unjust hospitalisation, and/or to ensure that those who need admission are admitted, even against their will. Changes in legislation are under consideration, and might include a clearer and more influential role for designated social workers. In many parts of the USA, it is the legal authorities who take the decision regarding compulsory admission, but the social work profession is nevertheless concerned to ensure that people's civil rights and liberties are protected. Because of the variation in procedure, the discussion of compulsory hospitalisation that follows looks at the decision-making process without specifying the roles of those involved: the issues raised are of significance to every social worker who is concerned about the treatment of the mentally ill.

The abuse of mental health legislation

In the history of psychiatry there have been some horrifying examples – some of them recent – of the misuse of psychiatric hospitalisation to 'falsely imprison' sane people. Although such events rarely come to light, it is right that social workers should have this concern at the forefront of their minds when considering the question of compulsory admission, especially when the pressure for admission comes from a person who might have something to gain from the 'patient' being removed. One obvious instance is when an elderly person shares his home with a married son or daughter. However, there have been reports of similar phenomena concerning residential staff and other non-relatives. For example, an elderly lady in a residential establishment was harassed, as well as being falsely described as mentally disturbed, in an apparent bid to gain possession of her flat for a member of the staff (Lund and Gardiner, 1977). A non-English-speaking couple, who accused the janitor of their building of theft, were committed to hospital after the janitor stated that they were insane (Kutner, 1962). Particular assessment problems can arise, in that the threat of being taken away against one's will, and the general commotion of a roomful of strangers, can trigger behaviour in a perfectly sane individual that could look like the symptoms of mental disorder – aggression, extreme distress, or stubborn silence.

Careful and impartial listening, and questioning of all the people involved, plus a determination to take things slowly and try to defuse the situation, may help to obtain a clearer view of what is going on. One source of useful evidence is information about relationships prior to this occasion. The National Schizophrenia Fellowship differs from other organisations concerned with mental health law in Britain in that it wants relatives' views to receive more, rather than less, recognition. It points to the many cases where a family's long and honourable record of tolerating difficult behaviour, while making enormous efforts to keep the patient out of hospital, is disregarded when in desperation they finally turn to the health or welfare services for assistance. The Fellowship urges that the request for hospitalisation be seen in the context of long periods of self-sacrifice on the family's part. Of course it is true that hard-pressed relatives have 'something to gain', in the sense of a respite from the burden they carry when the patient is at home; but their rights have to be taken into account as well. One interpretation of the criteria for involuntary admission is that the person is unable to care for himself: one might argue that it is unreasonable to take for granted the family's willingness to do the caring.

The problems of making an assessment on the basis of hearsay evidence, rather than observed behaviour, are well known. There can be no doubt that alarm on the informant's part can lead to an element of exaggeration, and in some families the belief that admission would be in the patient's best interests may colour the description of his behaviour that they give. However, before jumping to the conclusion that the person who now seems calm and reasonable could not possibly have been recently acting as he is reported to have done, we need to remember that even severe disturbance is not necessarily continuous. There can be long periods of apparent normality, interspersed with episodes of disordered behaviour. One man attended a dinner party and behaved exactly like his normal self, whereas beforehand he was muttering, shouting and threatening; soon after the meal he accused his host of homosexual rape. During those few 'normal' hours, even an experienced observer might have judged this person to be in absolutely no need of psychiatric treatment. Some patients, even when being interviewed by a skilled professional, can suppress delusional talk, and deny the existence of their symptoms. This is why other people's reports of recent behaviour must be taken into account. This said, if there are doubts about the veracity of the informant, the only solution is to spend more time in an attempt to clarify matters. Day care may provide an appropriate setting for a period of observation, or it may be possible to find another independent witness. In some cases, the patient may calm down, or accept sedation, and could be visited again a few hours later.

There are, of course, a number of other issues relating to the question of other people misrepresenting the situation in order to get the 'patient' committed to hospital. The foregoing discussion is intended, not to refute the views of civil-rights campaigners, but to try to redress the balance in this contentious area, and to suggest one or two practical safeguards.

Besides taking into account the (admittedly remote) possibility of a plot against the 'patient', it is necessary to consider three key questions: whether the patient ought to be admitted for his own safety; for the sake of his health; or for the protection of others.

Compulsory admission in practice

Dawson (1972) studied fifty cases of compulsory admission to a psychiatric hospital in London. Reasons for the decision included:

disturbed behaviour reported by others; public nuisance; socially embarrassing behaviour; predicted (rather than actual) social or family disruption or violence; and hardship to the family considered to be 'beyond the limits of what is ordinarily regarded as tolerable'. The investigators' judgement was that all but two of these admissions were fully justified; the other two were 'doubtful', and even in these cases there seemed to be no feasible alternative, since clarification of an ambiguous situation was essential. The main diagnostic groups concerned were schizophrenia, hypomania and severe depression. Clare (1979) describes what he calls a typical case for compulsory admission: the hypomanic businessman who was not at all aggressive, but who spent his family's savings and endangered his reputation and his job. Gordon (1978), reporting eight cases of compulsory admission, lists examples of hypomania, suicidal mood, severe delirium tremens, senile dementia, paranoid delusions and fire setting.

From these accounts of actual practice, it is clear that the terms used in the English Mental Health Act 1959 – 'health', 'safety', and 'the protection of other persons' – are open to varied interpretation, and that decisions taken are as much a matter of value judgement as of professional expertise. Many of the cases would certainly not satisfy the criteria proposed by Gostin (1975), that 'only grave and genuinely probable future harm to others should form the basis of compulsory admission and this prediction should be backed up by recent overt actions'. Clare's point, that practice challenges theory, seems a valid one (Clare, 1979). Bearing in mind the many ethical and definitional problems involved, it may still be worth tracing out some possible lines of thinking in relation to questions of health and safety.

Suicide and deliberate self-harm

The possibility of suicide or deliberate self-harm is a key question. Certain background variables have been regularly associated with a raised risk of suicide: elderly, male, divorced or widowed. Significant 'life events' include recent bereavement and becoming unemployed. Diagnostic categories carrying a particularly high risk are: depression (especially agitated depression, and depression accompanied by self-blame, insomnia, hypochondriasis or physical illness); personality disorder; addiction to drugs or alcohol (Stengel, 1973; Sainsbury, 1973). Attempted suicide – or, more accurately, deliberate self-harm with or without evidence of true suicidal intent – is particularly common among people in their late teens and early twenties (Morgan, 1979). The best predictive factor seems to be whether the person has made a previous suicidal attempt: in this case the risk is increased tenfold (Priest and Steinert, 1977).

However, careful interviewing is needed in order to assess the individual case. Talking about suicide is a very serious indicator – it must never be assumed to be a substitute for action. Some people drop hints: 'I won't be needing your help', 'They won't have to put up with me much longer', 'I won't be here for Christmas'; and it can even be done jokingly: 'I might just take a walk off the end of the pier.' Alternatively, the person intent on suicide may take steps to put his affairs in order. It is important, especially if the person appears depressed, to pursue the topic in quite a firm and dogged fashion: 'Do you sometimes wish you could end it all?', 'Have you thought about how you might do it?' (the more specific the planning the greater the risk). There is no justification for the view that such questioning encourages suicidal behaviour – unless of course the interviewer fails to show concern and willingness to help.

It is particularly important to discover the intentions of people who may be unwilling to talk about their self-destructive thoughts because they are ashamed; and to look for non-verbal as well as verbal responses to the questions.

The freedom to kill oneself is advocated by many who, like Szasz (1974), insist that to take over a person's responsibility for his own actions is to take away his human dignity, and in certain circumstances, such as when the person is suffering from an incurable and painful illness, it is difficult to argue against this view: the desire to kill oneself can be rational, and in no way related to mental disorder. However, in very many instances it may be possible to help someone to cope with a problem that he believes to be insoluble, and preventing him from taking his own life wins time for this to be attempted.

The person who is depressed is often basing his decision on a mistaken view of himself or his world, which will quickly dissipate as a result of treatment for the depression. Fox (1973) comments, 'One has yet to meet anyone who, on recovery, showed animosity. But one has met gratitude, and the comment "Why didn't somebody do something before?"' Wing (1978) suggests that the person ought to be helped through his current phase of depression and given another opportunity for choice: 'There is no way of stopping people from killing themselves if they really wish to do so.' A rather different line of argument is espoused by Altrocchi (1980), who devotes a section of his book to the severe problems of those who are bereaved by suicide, arguing that their rights ought to be safeguarded.

In some cases, it is suspected that the person's intention is not suicide, but non-fatal self-harm, usually on the rather dubious grounds that he has made 'suicidal gestures' in the past. This may well be the case, but the danger remains that on the next occasion either his intention might be more serious or he might kill himself by mistake. A client of the author's, who had taken no less than twenty small overdoses on previous occasions, took a massive and fatal overdose on the twenty-first. Sometimes this patient's behaviour resembled the type of 'manipulative crisis' described earlier (pp. 150–1); at other times her intentions were expressed only in veiled hints, or not revealed at all.

A smaller group, who may also be described as a 'danger to themselves', are those who mutilate themselves (Ross and McKay, 1979). Like the patients who make 'suicidal gestures', self-mutilators are often classified as 'psychopathic' or 'personality-disordered' Their behaviour is often described as 'attention-seeking' or manipulative, but it can often be equally well construed as a means of releasing severe tension.

The possibility that someone will injure himself either by a 'suicidal gesture' or by self-mutilation is a borderline category of conditions suggesting the need for compulsory admission on the grounds of danger to self. The results of such actions can be permanent and disfiguring (in the case of self-mutilation), or can cause physical or mental damage (in the case of overdoses), even if the person's life is not endangered. Against this, we have to weigh the consequences of depriving people of the opportunity to learn more positive ways of coping in the community.

Risk to health

The possibility that a person's health will suffer if he does not enter hospital arises in a number of circumstances in addition to those we have just considered. Patients with hypomania may continue to approach a state of mania, and in the process will become physically and mentally exhausted as well as suffering the effects of malnutrition; and those with depression may be unable to take care of their basic needs. The person with acute schizophrenia will become increasingly disturbed, and some authorities suggest that if treatment is delayed the degree of handicap later on will be more severe than it need have been (Priest and Woolfson, 1978). In the case of chronic and progressive organic disorders, damage to health may result through neglect of safety precautions, hygiene or diet.

The criterion of 'endangered health' can also encompass almost any form of abnormal behaviour or self-neglect that is likely to have painful repercussions for the patient. Clare's (1979) businessman would suffer great distress when he realised the harm he had done to himself and his family during his hypomanic phase; socially embarrassing behaviour, or behaviour likely to disrupt personal relationships, could also fit a somewhat stretched definition of danger to health. Indeed, it seems that many psychiatrists, social workers and relatives employ an extremely broad definition of 'danger to health', and they simply weigh the disadvantages to the patient of being forced to enter hospital, against the disadvantages of staying in the community. The stricter the legal definitions, the less opportunity for others to make this choice on the patient's behalf. We do not know how many patients benefit and how many lose thereby.

The protection of others

Some of the indicators of danger to others parallel those of danger to self. For example, the depressed mother may believe that her children, as well as she herself, would be better off dead. The deluded schizophrenic patient may feel obliged to defend himself against his persecutors, or his voices may order him to attack other people. The hypomanic patient may become irascible if he is frustrated, and his distraught family cannot be expected to refrain from trying to control his behaviour.

Prins (1975) gives a number of case examples where warnings from the patient himself had preceded acts of aggression. The warnings included straightforward verbal threats, writings full of paranoid or sadistic references, and incidents of cruelty to animals. It is not known what proportion of such warnings are actually followed by overt violence, but Prins makes a good case for enquiry along these lines, and for taking the information very seriously. However, research on the prediction of violence has shown that the number of 'false positives' (wrong predictions in the direction of overestimating the probability of violence) is invariably greater than the number of correct predictions (Monahan, 1975). In fact, violence among psychiatric patients is extremely rare. It is a matter for value judgement whether it is considered that even a remote risk is grounds for compulsory admission, and those making such decisions will be influenced both by their assessment of the benefits or otherwise of hospital care, and by the 'climate of the times' – public opinion swings back and forth on this issue, and is often an unacknowledged determinant of the actions of both judges and mental health professionals.

While any general discussion of the dilemmas faced by those involved in deciding about compulsory admission is open to criticism for 'fence sitting', it has to be accepted that in practice there is a responsibility to take decisions, even in the context of inadequate knowledge. If the compulsory admission was an error, then the cost is to be borne in terms of stigma, with possibly long-term and serious consequences, lowered self-esteem and loss of liberty; if allowing the person to remain at home was an error, then the cost may be illness, or other consequences of self-destructive behaviour: the stigma that undoubtedly attaches to those who behave oddly in the community, embarrassment, and perhaps guilt, and possibly harm or distress to other people. We have to weigh the results of an error in either direction, and be aware that an ethical choice is being made. If more alternatives to hospital were available (day-centres, hostels, crisis intervention services), many of the patients admitted against their will, and many who receive inadequate care in the community, might be better served, and the choice between hospital and community would not confront us so starkly. Meanwhile, the best we can hope for is that those of us who share the responsibility for this decision remind ourselves constantly of the consequences of our decision, and remain fully aware of the limitations of our ability to assess and predict.

Crisis intervention

Among the most frequently proposed alternatives to hospitalisation is crisis intervention. Parad (1976) emphasises its value in terms of both reduction of distress and financial savings, and others have claimed that it can prevent, as well as alleviate, mental illness (for example, Caplan, 1964).

Although the general principles of crisis intervention are familiar to mental health professionals, especially to social workers, it is more often preached than it is practised. Clarke (1971), reporting on the work of mental welfare officers called to psychiatric emergencies, notes that they did little in the way of constructive family intervention, apart from assessing the need for admission to hospital; and the paper by Gleisner, Hewett and Mann (1972) includes the observation that some of the patients admitted to hospital were reacting to a social or domestic problem. Olsen (1979b) comments that crisis intervention is not given sufficient attention in relation to mental health emergencies; but the truth of this observation is obscured by the frequent misuse of the term – sometimes this looks suspiciously like a cover-up for providing only 'band-aid' work with problems that arouse considerable anxiety.

Crisis intervention as a theory of behaviour derives from psychoanalytic ego psychology. At the risk of oversimplification, its chief tenets can be summarised as follows. A crisis is defined as 'an upset in the steady state', when the individual is faced with an obstacle to important life-goals, and cannot overcome it by means of his customary methods of problem-solving. A crisis is a state of affairs precipitated by a stressor event – a combination of objective reality, the person's own definition of the event, his level of perceptual and coping capacity, and the resources available to him at the time. At crisis there is a break in normal functioning. It is a turning point or testing point. It can lead either to 'breakdown', or to personality growth and increased competence. Rapoport (1962), drawing on the work of Gerald Caplan, proposes that a crisis has three or four phases: (1) a rise in tension; habitual problem-solving mechanisms are evoked in an effort to preserve the 'steady state'; (2) a further rise in tension; disorganisation of normal behaviour; feelings of distress and helplessness; the person may try to avoid action or may make desperate-seeming attempts to solve the problem; (3)

mobilisation of resources; the problem may be redefined; a solution of some sort is reached; the solution may be successful, incomplete or maladaptive. It is suggested that this process lasts no more than six weeks. In some cases, a fourth phase occurs: there is a major disorganisation of personality and behaviour; 'nervous breakdown', perhaps with psychotic symptoms.

It is proposed that the optimum time for intervention is the second – 'distress and helplessness' – phase. At this point, the defences are loosened, motivation is at its peak, and the person is responsive to the possibility of change and to the influence of those who offer help.

Rapoport (1970) outlines the main components of crisis intervention as an approach to treatment. The chief distinguishing feature is the timing: it is crucial to reach the client at the height of his distress, and before a possibly maladaptive resolution of the crisis can take place, further, it is suggested that help should be concentrated within a short period of time. Assessment is rapid, and focuses on the 'presenting problem', and on positive resources within the person and in his environment. The treatment procedures are not clearly laid down, but they usually include helping the client to gain a cognitive grasp of his situation, and selecting specific and limited goals, and also tasks for him to undertake. The worker is more active than in long-term psychodynamic treatment, but the client also is encouraged to take action on his own behalf. Family members are often involved, and the client remains in the community if at all possible.

Although the rationale for these elements of the crisis intervention treatment package derives from the crisis intervention theory of behaviour, powerful arguments can also be advanced on the basis of research in other fields of work, for example evaluations of time-limited and task-centred treatment, of family therapy and of behaviour modification. In considering the application of crisis intervention in a psychiatric emergency, we have first to assess how well the model fits the individual case. As was suggested at the beginning of this chapter, stressful situations where psychiatric disorder is not to the forefront – for example, the family who have received upsetting news – can very readily be construed in a crisis framework. Where psychiatric disturbance is clearly a reaction to recent stress – the acute anxiety state, the 'reactive' depression, or the so-called 'psychogenic psychosis' (acute symptoms that quickly subside if the person is admitted) – then immediate, structured, short-term help seems theoretically and pragmatically appropriate, if the intervention can be timed to begin before the client's disturbance has gone beyond the 'distress and helplessness' stage. One difficulty arising from this analysis is that many manifestations of mental disorder coming to the attention of the crisis team have indeed passed this stage, and the patient is already in stage four, 'breakdown'. Many people who have severe, acute symptoms may have shown little sign of passing through the stages described in the crisis model, and indeed have no obvious 'insurmountable obstacle to life goals' for the team to assist with: the situation simply does not fit the model.

If, on the other hand, we turn our attention to the family as a whole, it becomes clear that the crisis model can very readily be applied to family members other than the designated patient, and crisis intervention procedures could do much to help them. They have experienced a stressor event (the patient's illness), and have not been able to cope with it without outside help; they may have had a period of turmoil while trying to deny or redefine the problem; and they may, if not given some timely assistance, solve the problem for themselves in one of a number of maladaptive ways: rejecting the patient as mad or bad, becoming over-protective, trying to deny that anything untoward has occurred, or finding a comforting but unconstructive 'explanation'. Two families of severely ill schizophrenic patients illustrate this type of maladaptive solution: one couple began making efforts to find friends for their daughter, claiming that her illness was 'just due to loneliness'; another couple said their son was 'mentally handicapped' because of a childhood accident. At the time of acute distress it might be possible to help such families to gain a clearer picture of the situation, and to plan a more constructive way of coping in the future.

These observations concerning the clients and situations that seem to fit the crisis model are borne out by an examination of accounts of crisis intervention in practice. Studies of crisis intervention programmes suggest that they are effective on a variety of measures. Decker and Stubblebine (1972) found that the crisis intervention team achieved a reduction in time spent in hospital, without increased readmission rates or increased need for welfare support in the community. Langsley *et al.* (1969, 1971) found that their crisis intervention group did at least as well on measures of social functioning, and were significantly less likely to be admitted or readmitted, than the control group who received ordinary hospital care. Gibbons *et al.* (1978), who provided task-centred, 'crisis-oriented' casework for overdose patients, found more change on measures of social problems, and greater satisfaction with the service, among the experimental group, as compared with the control group, who received routine follow-up.

However, it is important to note that most of the programmes that have been reported are either limited to those 'patients' who are facing a 'problem in living' and suffering an acute reaction to a family or social problem, or include types of intervention not usually emphasised in the crisis intervention literature. It is unfortunate that, so often, the accounts in the social work literature read as though almost any psychiatric emergency can be dealt with by the immediate offer of short-term psychological or social help. For this reason it is important to stress the limitations of 'classical' crisis intervention, and, by implication, the limitations of the social worker who answers an emergency call with his mind fixed upon crisis intervention. First, consider the question of treatment. Decker and Stubblebine's successful programme was in fact with patients who entered hospital (Decker and Stubblebine, 1972). In Langsley and Kaplan's book (1968) there are many instances of the use of medication on a long-term basis, and of intensive supervision in the community. Second, consider the question of which client groups are likely to benefit from crisis intervention. One aspect of the Langsley *et al.* studies, which is often omitted from second-hand accounts of their findings, is that all their clients were voluntary patients and living with relatives. The Gibbons *et al.* (1978) study excluded clients considered to require, or already receiving, psychiatric treatment. All these workers accept that crisis intervention is not a universal remedy and must be applied with discrimination.

Flomenhaft and Langsley (1971) comment that crisis intervention had little effect on long-term problems of individual and family behaviour, and that about half their sample needed long-term help. In other words, crisis intervention is not an alternative to extended community care and treatment. Ewing (1978) gives some further contra-indications: intoxication; severe agitation; the possibility of deliberate self-harm; inability to talk openly and coherently, to think clearly, to perceive reality – in general terms, being unwilling or unable to undertake the work that crisis intervention demands.

If we include under crisis intervention voluntary and compulsory hospital admission, and medical treatment (indeed any type of help so long as it is given promptly), we are surely stretching a technical term beyond the limits of its usefulness. We must accept that crisis intervention as it is usually understood is only one of a number of services that ought to be available for those who need urgent help.

14

Social Work in Hospital

As we have seen, a crisis intervention service may obviate the need for hospital admission for some acutely disturbed people. Facilities such as day-centres, day-hospitals and hostels can make it possible for people to get assessment treatment or support without being cut off from all aspects of ordinary life. But some psychiatric patients need the surveillance, respite from stress and responsibilities, and intensive treatment that only an in-patient facility can provide. Without underestimating the risk of institutionalism, we should remember that many modern psychiatric wards bear little resemblance to the state hospitals described by Goffman (1961), and that stigmatisation can be as much a consequence of odd behaviour in the community as of mental hospital admission. The social worker can contribute in helping to reduce the ill effects, and maximise the benefits of hospital care. This chapter considers some aspects of social work that relate specifically to the psychiatric in-patient, and concludes with a brief discussion of the question of a hospital base for the specialist psychiatric social worker.

When patients are having intensive medical treatment the social worker may have little contact with them, but may nevertheless be in touch with the family. Although this is more often the province of the nursing staff, the social worker too may find it necessary to act as a link-person between family and medical staff, perhaps explaining the treatment procedures, the psychiatrist's plans, or the hospital's rules and routines. He may also be entrusted with messages to the psychiatrist: questions about prognosis, about how best to cope, and requests for an interview. It is a sad reflection on our services that families often feel excluded and bewildered, and too nervous of 'authority' to put their concerns to the appropriate staff member direct. Social workers, although willing to act as a go-between in such circumstances, might also seek to relieve themselves of this particular job by trying to change hospital practice, so that doctors become more approachable, and also more skilled in the task that social workers often have to become adept at: explaining 'medical matters' in language that people with no specialist knowledge can understand. This is one of the areas that can be profitably tackled by a relatives' group. Such groups have been set up in many places, often with the backing of a social worker, and they can use their pooled experience and influence to cope with problems that are beyond the capacity of any individual family.

The other important linking role is between patient and family. Relationships often become strained at the point of admission. The essential skill is in helping people talk to each other. Through diplomatic message-carrying, and tactful chairing of family conferences, one can do much to help relatives deal with anger or anxiety about the patient's behaviour, and to clear up misunderstandings on both sides. Hospital admission often constitutes a crisis point at which unresolved family difficulties – not necessarily related to the patient's illness – may come to a head, and become amenable to a problem-solving endeavour. In the section on crisis intervention it was suggested that it may be appropriate to construe hospital admission in these terms. In some cases, the patient's problems have been 'accommodated' by the family for years, but in a manner that has done little to ensure that he has had appropriate support, or even medical attention. Sampson, Messinger and Towne (1965) found examples of near-neglect stretching back over several years, and its converse, over-involvement and taking over the person's normal role – patterns which only came to light at the time of admission. In these circumstances, admission offers an opportunity for re-thinking the family life-style with help from a social worker.

In the case of the longer-stay patient, the social worker, besides sharing with other professionals in the tasks of rehabilitation into work and accommodation, has a special role with regard to rehabilitation into family and social relationships.

Where family ties have suffered, it may be possible to re-establish relationships. A structured approach to this task was developed by O'Brien and Azrin (1973). Relatives received formal, specific invitations to come to the ward, and were assisted with transport. Every effort was made to ensure that the occasion was reinforcing for the visitor, and it was clearly spelled out that the visit could be terminated at any time if the relative so wished. Visits by the patient to the relative were also carefully organised. Much planning went into how the time together would be spent, and the patients were given behavioural training in ways of making the occasion as pleasant as possible, for example by preparing refreshments and making interesting conversation. O'Brien and Azrin achieved remarkable success in bringing together people who had been estranged for many years, and made it possible to discharge the patients back to their families. Other workers, in a geriatric setting, helped patients to establish the practice of letter-writing and, as a result of the project, significantly increased the number of letters the patients received (Goldstein and Baer, 1976).

Whether or not such help in re-establishing relationships is part of preparation for discharge, encouraging family and other social contacts and visits outside hospital forms part of a series of tasks that come under the general heading of 'normalisation'. Social workers, with their local knowledge, and their familiarity with many aspects of people's lives that may be overlooked in the hospital's concentration on people in their patient-role, are aware of the normal responsibilities and satisfactions of which long-stay patients may quite unnecessarily be deprived. Along with other professionals, especially, perhaps, occupational therapists, the social worker should be constantly seeking ways in which the in-patient can live a life like that of any other member of society: travelling on public transport, spending money in shops, going to pubs and cinemas. Many long-stay patients have 'forgotten' how to do these things, so it is not merely a matter of pointing out opportunities, or even arranging them on the patients' behalf. Helping someone who has lost confidence, or lacks the necessary abilities, is a task that requires a great deal of patience, sensitivity and skill.

The author remembers a group of elderly ladies who reacted with both anxiety and annoyance at the suggestion that they might take a trip to the town centre. Closer enquiry revealed that they not only feared the bus journey, but they were unsure about the procedure for going into a shop and choosing new clothes. Furthermore, they were alarmed that this suggestion might be the thin end of the wedge – the start of a programme leading to discharge! In this situation, it was possible to assure them that nobody would be discharged against her will, and they were then happy to co-operate in a programme of learning to undertake more and more everyday activities outside the hospital. The example of these ladies is a poignant reminder of how a mental hospital can become the only home that the person has or wants. Braginsky and his colleagues (1969) gave a striking demonstration of a similar phenomenon: patients who believed they were being assessed with a view to discharge reported serious symptoms, in an obvious effort to discourage the psychiatrist from recommending discharge. In another experiment, chronic patients (unlike recently admitted patients) biased their answers on a questionnaire to give an impression of mental disturbance. The solution to this problem lies not in the hospital itself, but in society's provision for people who need a haven. As Williams (1971) expresses it:

> Increasingly, the mental hospital is becoming the only place where a person can obtain food, a roof over his head, without paying or working. Hardly surprising, then, that those who cannot get such necessities in the world outside, are prepared to tell a few little lies about what is happening inside their heads, in order to gain access to this service.

For some long-stay patients, it may be the friendships they have formed that are the key reason for their desire to remain in hospital: the 'home' as much as the haven. Some of the facilities mentioned in Chapter 12 might meet these patients' needs, especially if they can be discharged as a group of friends, or else helped to maintain their links at the hospital after they have left.

Although the number of long-stay patients is gradually being reduced, it is unlikely that this trend will go on indefinitely, unless there is a very great increase in alternative sheltered accommodation. This means that the kinds of help summarised as rehabilitation and normalisation will continue to be required.

In-patients also need help with a variety of legal and practical problems of a highly specialised nature, some of which are appropriately the concern of the social worker. For example, those who are detained involuntarily may need advice about the provisions for appeal, and appeals tribunals can involve the social worker in either a decision-making role, or as an informant or expert witness, providing reports on family and community resources. Questions concerning the need for power of attorney, or a guardianship order, or the making of wills, also have a strong social element. The patient's financial benefits and earnings from work in hospital can require specialist attention.

Another important aspect of hospital social work is the ability to work at the level of the organisation itself. Social workers with a 'systems' orientation have worked to change policies on general wards; and similarly in psychiatry, problems experienced by a number of patients and/or their families may need to be approached at ward or management level. Examples from the author's experience include the question of visiting hours, use of a patients' canteen, and administrative barriers to co-operation with a voluntary agency for problem drinkers. In order to tackle such matters in a rational and non-piecemeal fashion, the worker needs knowledge of organisational structures in general, plus special knowledge of his own hospital in particular. Cumming and Cumming (1957) describe their study of a large state hospital as a social system, and how an accurate understanding of the organisation enabled them to work towards changes affecting many of its patients and staff. The present-day social worker, confronted with a less daunting institution, and pursuing less ambitious goals, can still learn from their analysis and their strategies.

I think the range of specialist knowledge and concentrated experience needed for the performance of the roles outlined here is sufficient to justify the continued existence of the hospital-based psychiatric social worker. A hospital base provides the opportunity to develop expertise. It also facilitates the close working relationship with other members of the inter-disciplinary team that is essential in providing co-ordinated, comprehensive help to both short- and long-stay patients. But being hospital-based also carries the risk of losing some of the very qualities that make the social worker's contribution so valuable: awareness of things social, knowledge of ordinary life and resources in the community. However, this is by no means an inevitable consequence, and the hospital social worker can and should follow up patients when they leave, visit their homes, and liaise closely with social work colleagues in the community, as well as with other services. Community-based colleagues have every right to complain if these tasks are omitted, and if the hospital social worker is seen to pass on the less promising, that is, chronic clients, and to take on an exclusively therapist role, leaving the other social work responsibilities to them.

The division of labour between hospital and community social workers will depend on a variety of considerations. Apart from obvious restrictions, such as distance from clients' homes, it is often proposed that the short-stay, and the 'revolving door' clients, are better served by social workers based outside hospital. On the other hand, it can be argued just as strongly that the client with repeated admissions may benefit from having a hospital social worker who gets to know him well. This debate continues, and each area tends to develop its own patterns of social work service. One thing is clear, however: opportunities for mutual consultation and close liaison must be built into the system. And it is the author's view that even if 'hospital specialism' can be done without, 'mental illness specialism' is essential.

15

Concluding Remarks: Research and Recording

Reading research does not seem to be as prominent an activity as it might be among practising social workers. Doing research is often viewed as a sophisticated luxury, reserved for members of other professions and those who are comfortably remote from the harsh realities of practice. Of course, it can be argued that social work with the mentally disordered is in no greater need of research-mindedness than any other aspect of social work; but if we are committed to trying to improve our service to this client group, we need to challenge the current state of affairs.

A great deal of excellent research has been done in psychiatry over recent years, and this book mentions only a small proportion of the findings that can enhance our practice now. Research is proceeding apace, so that everyone who works in this field needs to try to keep abreast of new information as it becomes available, by reading the journals and attending conferences. It is important to go to the sources: second-hand accounts (this book is no exception!) tend to highlight those facets of other people's work that best support the particular bias of the author. This is why, for example, it is not uncommon for social workers to expect more of crisis intervention than it can possibly deliver. In this case the problem is largely due to incomplete second-hand reports of the studies. The view that parents cause schizophrenia is still widely held among social workers: this is due to the uncritical acceptance of defective research.

None of us is immune from such failings. Not only must we read more, we must also read more critically. Fischer (1978) has proposed a helpful set of guidelines for assessing the value of research studies; and Sheldon (1978) suggests that we need to discard much that is speculative if we are not to be overburdened with conflicting theories that have neither empirical validity nor practical usefulness. Writing as a social work teacher, I am aware that it is one of the academic's paid responsibilities to undertake this work, and that field social workers in most agencies are not permitted the time they require to fulfil this part of their professional (ethical) obligations. However, the more of us that are concerned about the proper understanding and dissemination of research, the faster we shall progress towards an approach to intervention with a sound supporting rationale.

The work on institutionalism (Wing and Brown, 1970), on depression in housewives (Brown and Harris, 1978), and on schizophrenia and family interaction (Vaughn and Leff, 1976), are examples of complex research studies that have yielded suggestions for service-planning and for individual casework as well. By contrast, intervention with a very small group of patients and families who had become estranged has been described and evaluated in painstaking detail (O'Brien and Azrin, 1973). This paper provides practical guidelines for our work with similar problems. Evaluative research on the treatment of phobias has been sufficiently rigorous and convincing for us to know what approach is most likely to help most patients (Marks, 1978). The dossier prepared by MIND (1978) on discrimination at work has done much to make policy-makers aware of the problem, and to encourage debate about how this form of injustice can be combated.

Knowing about studies like these is useful in our day-to-day work with individuals, families and small groups, and such knowledge is vital if social workers are to influence the provision of services, whether within one's own small working group, in local drives to get resources and alter the way things are currently done, or in a national campaign to change the law or to obtain better state provision for the mentally disordered. We have to be armed not only with arguments, but also with facts. If we believe that it is part of our responsibility to seek change at any level, then it is a matter of professional ethics to keep up with research.

Despite the advances in knowledge referred to throughout this book, there remain large areas of ignorance. We still know very little about the nature of mental disorder, and in many situations deciding how best to help is a matter of intuition rather than of rational choice. Social work as a profession has a duty to add its contribution to the general store of knowledge that will sooner or later lead to more humane and more effective services. Studies carried out by Olsen (1976a) on boarding-out, by Ryan and Hewett (1976) on hostels, and by Creer (Creer and Wing, 1974) on living with schizophrenia, are outstanding examples of research contributions by social workers.

Research, after all, is no more and no less than purposeful, systematic knowledge-gathering. If we define it like this, it becomes clear that 'doing research' is something that can be built into the daily activities of the field social worker. The rest of this chapter outlines some possibilities.

Information about resources and needs

The social work practitioner, especially if he has a caseload composed largely of psychiatric patients and their families, is in a unique position to amass the sorts of knowledge that could influence the services these clients receive. But this knowledge is unsystematic, impressionistic, and rarely put to use by anyone except that worker himself with his own clients. Let us consider some examples of important knowledge areas.

A frequent type of referral is the request to place a client in a day-centre. The worker soon becomes aware that finding a place at all is difficult, and that some centres are either hard to get to (a transport problem), or unwilling to accept certain clients (a matching problem). In such circumstances, it is understandable that the worker may omit to record his client's need and the reason why he has not taken steps to meet it – or else the information is buried in the individual file. Yet this social worker could gather together evidence of needs and resources that might lead to an improvement in provision within the region. The 'non-researching' – or non-recording – social worker could certainly, if asked, give his opinion about the situation; but the worker with facts and figures is in a far better position to contribute to planning, and to exert pressure on the controllers of resources – his own agency, or perhaps a voluntary body that might finance new facilities if the need were brought to its attention. It has been shown that in some areas hostels for 'short-term rehabilitation' are under-used, whereas large numbers of patients with little hope of returning to work in the foreseeable future are homeless: facts – not impressions – about this state of affairs have led to reconsideration of the aims of the hostels. Certain hostels may consistently refuse to take patients on maintenance medication, such as lithium carbonate or phenothiazines. Where this is shown to be a recurring pattern, the social worker and his colleagues might plan a discussion with the hostel staff in the hope of achieving a change in their policy.

Another example of a subject area of considerable concern to the mentally disordered and their families is that of welfare rights. Such bodies as the National Schizophrenia Fellowship collate information on the experiences of claimants, and disseminate it for the benefit of others who are in difficulty, as well as using it to support their arguments for policy changes at national and local level. The social worker can both add to the fund of knowledge by providing details of experience in his own area, and himself collate it in order to seek a change in procedure at the local social security office. We have to accept that an account of a single case, though it can sometimes be persuasive, may be disregarded as a one-off event.

Investigators running large-scale research studies often hold feedback sessions for the people who have provided their data. In the same way, small-scale research on resources for the mentally ill can be accompanied by feedback to the people who provide the facilities – for example, day-centre and hostel staff and managers – and, equally important, to bodies who are not fulfilling a particular need, or have withdrawn a needed resource. Both negative and positive feedback are valuable – too often, only the negative feedback is given, the successful efforts by workers and managers being taken for granted. A valuable spin-off of feedback procedures is that they can become mutual. The hostel warden, the day-centre staff, and the social security officers can inform the social worker about such matters as appropriateness of referrals and quality of back-up support, and can provide extra detail about the clients' fortunes.

How and where to record all the diverse facts about needs and resources is a major problem for the busy social worker trying to keep his records up-to-date. This problem means that much potentially useful information is well-nigh impossible to retrieve. While there are certainly no easy solutions, one useful approach is to keep a running record with 'hard' data separately from the 'softer' data of our casework assessment and procedures. Lavan (1980) describes a method of recording on punch-cards, which makes it possible for large amounts of information to be retrieved and collated.

Alternatively, information can be recorded by facility as well as by case. Most social work offices maintain resource files, but these tend to give a rather static account of the facility. A brief, running record of the experiences of social workers and their clients in using, or seeking to use, a particular facility provides information that is readily accessible to colleagues, and can yield feedback for the providers of the resource and evidence to back up efforts to secure improvements. Over time, the record will help to clarify the impression that, for example, Hostel X has staff who go to considerable lengths to accommodate phases of bizarre or withdrawn behaviour, or Hostel Y is particularly successful in obtaining work opportunities for its residents.

It might be argued that the task of gathering information of the kind discussed here belongs properly to the role of the designated research officer or the administrator. However, the social worker on the front line has special opportunities and responsibilities. In collaboration with colleagues in his own agency, and with members of his other team, the multi-disciplinary team, he can work towards improvements in the services for his current and future clients, and for many other people as well.

Effectiveness research

Researchers studying the work of social workers (Goldberg and Warburton, 1979) have developed a particular style of record-keeping, the 'case review system'. The worker lists the problems to be resolved at the beginning of intervention, and action taken and planned; and at intervals returns to this check-list to record progress and future plans. Similarly, in psychiatry, along with other medical specialties, the 'problem-oriented' case record is gaining acceptance (Fry, 1978). Looking at these developments with an awareness of the immense difficulties involved in trying to evaluate psycho-social interventions, one cannot but feel that such systems are still very far from providing real evidence about the effectiveness or otherwise of our work. Nevertheless, compared with traditional narrative forms of recording they offer considerable advantages. At the very least, we are constrained to state in advance what we hope to achieve by the particular actions we are taking, and to note whether or not our objectives have been met. This does not, of course, provide definite proof that our intervention was responsible for the outcome.

However, if a series of clients do well at job interviews following social skills training, whereas clients who receive only general advice about job-finding do less well, then we have at least some support for the view that social skills training might be useful for similar clients with similar needs. That information will be useful for the training officer who is considering whether funds should be allocated to teaching social workers how to conduct social skills groups. In a tentative way, innumerable questions about methods of intervention can be elucidated. And even where the intervention is hard to classify, and the client or his problem unusual, the social worker who keeps a problem-oriented record will be monitoring his own work, and will at least be able to recognise whether his help is proving ineffectual, and whether he ought to change tack.

Better evidence, though still only suggestive, is obtained by the more detailed single-case design (Jayaratne and Levy, 1979; Sheldon, 1978). This type of practice research, mainly done by behavioural workers, requires that the problem be specified precisely, and expressed in terms of a baseline. This is a rating or measurement of the behaviour, feelings or thoughts that are causing problems when the social worker begins his intervention. It is repeated at intervals, in order to monitor progress. This is the basic 'before-during-after' design. More sophisticated designs are available, which offer stronger evidence that the intervention is in fact responsible for any change that occurs. Besides measurements of the frequency of a concrete, observable behaviour, simple rating scales can be used by either worker or client, to assess change in feelings or attitudes.

Even where a sophisticated single-case design provides very powerful evidence that the procedures used are in fact having a beneficial effect, this does not permit us to assume that the next person who comes along is going to benefit from the same procedures: in other words, it is not possible to generalise from a single case, no matter how sure we are that what we did in that case was helpful. However, if we test our procedure out repeatedly in this way, then we can build up a powerful rationale for trying the same approach with the next client who presents a similar set of difficulties. The author has used the single-case design with a wide variety of problem areas: getting up in the morning, doing household chores, delusional talk, eating, reaction to teasing, sexual activity, rows, feelings of depression. In all such problems we need to specify the behaviour exactly, and count its incidence, or else use a rating scale – for example, of anxiety level or depressed mood.

Problems of an 'either–or' variety, such as getting a job, finding accommodation, or obtaining social security benefit, clearly do not require this type of monitoring: either the objective has been met or it has not. However, it is not unusual for us to treat a 'frequency' or 'intensity' problem as if it were an 'either–or' problem. Examples include budgeting: this is not a one-off problem, but will probably change gradually, with ups and downs along the way. Similarly, one talk with the family about the importance of taking medication might indeed have the effect that the patient takes it consistently thereafter, but it is more likely that the situation will require careful monitoring. Attendance at a day-centre, reducing the frequency of family rows, overcoming agoraphobia, are further examples of objectives that are not 'either–or'.

The kind of very small-scale, outcome-oriented research outlined here is within the capabilities of every social work practitioner: 'building research into practice', as Fischer (1978) calls it, will provide a basis for large-scale evaluative studies, which should come after hypotheses about 'what helps' have been tested out repeatedly by many different social workers in many settings.

Most of the research quoted in this book comes from the efforts of workers trained in other disciplines. Some of them are academics in the fields of psychology, sociology or social administration. But others are practitioners, especially psychiatrists – the relatively new specialism of community psychiatry has provided us with much useful information – and also clinical psychologists, who have contributed to our knowledge of treatment procedures, and given us new research tools, such as the single-case design.

Social workers have much to gain by becoming more attentive to the findings of other workers. But there is another side to the matter: social workers can bring a unique perspective to bear on the problems of the mentally disordered and their families. This means that besides reading the research reports from other professionals, we ought to be able to comment upon them helpfully; and besides reading research, we ought to be doing it. And so, like many commentators before me, I end with a plea for research – not as an alternative to social action or 'simply doing the job', but as a prerequisite for better campaigning and more responsible practice. In the words of the Seebohm Committee (1968):

> The Personal Social Services are large-scale experiments in ways of helping where there is a need. It is both wasteful and irresponsible to set experiments in motion and to omit to record and analyse what happens. It makes no sense in terms of administrative efficiency, and however little intended, it indicates a careless attitude towards human welfare.

Appendix A: Suggestions for Further Reading

General psychiatry

Meacher, Mollie (ed.) (1979) *New Methods in Mental Health Care*, Pergamon, Oxford.

Priest, R. G. and Steinert, J. (1977) *Insanity: A Study of Major Psychiatric Disorders*, Macdonald & Evans, London.

Priest, R. G. and Woolfson, G. (1978) *Minski's Handbook of Psychiatry*, 7th edn, Heinemann, London.

Stafford-Clark, D. and Smith, A. C. (1978) *Psychiatry for Students*, 5th edn, Heinemann, London.

Willis, J. (1976) *Clinical Psychiatry*, Blackwell, Oxford.

Social work and mental disorder

Olsen, M. Rolf (ed.) (1976) *Differential Approaches in Social Work with the Mentally Disordered*, BASW, Birmingham.

Social and philosophical issues

Clare, A. (1976) *Psychiatry in Dissent*, Tavistock, London.

Gostin, L. (1975) *The Mental Health Act from 1959 to 1975, Vol. 1: A MIND Special Report*, MIND (National Association for Mental Health), London.

Miles, A. (1981) *The Mentally Ill in Contemporary Society*, Martin Robertson, London.

Scheff, T. J. (ed.) (1967) *Mental Illness and Social Processes*, Harper & Row, New York.

Wing, J. K. (1978) *Reasoning about Madness*, Oxford University Press, Oxford.

Schizophrenia

Rollins, H. R. (ed.) (1980) *Coping with Schizophrenia*, National Schizophrenia Fellowship, London.
Wing, J. K. (ed.) (1978) *Schizophrenia: Towards a New Synthesis*, Academic Press, London.

Depression, grief and suicide

Clare, A. (1980) 'The Treatment of Depression' in Tennant, G. (ed.), *Current Trends in Treatment in Psychiatry*, Pitman, London.
McAuley, R. (1980) 'Commentary on Current Trends in the Treatment of Depression' in Tennant, G. (ed.), *Current Trends in Treatment in Psychiatry*, Pitman, London.
Parkes, C. M. (1972) *Bereavement*, Tavistock, London.
Priest, R. G. (1977) 'The Affective Psychoses' in Priest, R. G. and Steinert, J., *Insanity: A Study of Major Psychiatric Disorders*, Macdonald & Evans, London.
Stengel, E. (1973) *Suicide and Attempted Suicide*, rev. edn, Penguin, Harmondsworth.

Neurotic disorders

Marks, I. M. (1973) 'Research in Neurosis: A Selective Review: 1 Causes and Courses', *Psychological Medicine*, 3, 436.
Marks, I. M. (1974) 'Research in Neurosis: A Selective Review: 2 Treatment', *Psychological Medicine*, 4, 1, pp. 89–109.
Rycroft, C. (1970) *Anxiety and Neurosis*, Penguin, Harmondsworth.

Personality disorder

Gunn, J. (1976) 'The Treatment of Psychopaths', in Gaind, R. and Hudson, B. L. (eds), *Current Themes in Psychiatry I*, Macmillan, London.
Prins, H. (1980) *Offenders, Deviants, or Patients?*, Tavistock, London.
Whiteley, J. S. (1970) 'The Psychopath and his Treatment' *British Journal of Hospital Medicine*, February, p. 263, reprinted in Silverstone, T. and Barraclough, B. (eds) (1975) *Contemporary Psychiatry*, Royal College of Psychiatrists, London.

Alcohol and drug abuse

Cook, T. (1975) *Vagrant Alcoholics*, Routledge & Kegan Paul, London.
Madden, J. S. (1979) *A Guide to Alcohol and Drug Dependence*, Wright, Bristol.

Orford, J. and Harwin, J. (eds) (1981) *Alcohol and the Family*, Croom Helm, London.

The elderly

Gray, B. and Isaacs, B. (1979) *Care of the Elderly Mentally Infirm*, Tavistock, London.
MIND (1979) *Positive Approaches to Mental Infirmity in Elderly People* (Report), National Association for Mental Health, London.

Organic disorders

Priest, R. and Steinert, J. (1977) *Insanity*, Macdonald & Evans, London, chs 2–6.

Children

Rutter, M. (1966) *Children of Sick Parents: an Environmental and Psychiatric Study*, Maudsley Monograph No. 16, Oxford University Press, Oxford.

Rehabilitation

Bennett, D. M. and Watts, F. N. (eds) (1982) *Principles of Psychiatric Rehabilitation*, Wiley, Chichester.
Olsen, M. R. (ed.) (1979) *The Care of the Mentally Disordered: an examination of some alternatives to hospital care*, BASW, Birmingham.
Wansbrough N. and Cooper, P. (1980) *Open Employment after Mental Illness*, Tavistock, London.
Wing, J. K. and Olsen, M. R. (eds) (1979) *Community Care for the Mentally Disabled*, Oxford University Press, Oxford.

Residential treatment

Ayllon, T. and Azrin, N. H. (1968) *The Token Economy*, Appleton-Century-Crofts, New York.
Hinshelwood, R. D. and Manning, N. (eds) (1979) *Therapeutic Communities*, Routledge & Kegan Paul, London.

Behaviour therapy

Stern, R. S. (1978) *Behavioural Techniques*, Academic Press, London.

Group therapy

Trower, P., Bryant, B. and Argyle, M. (eds) (1978) *Social Skills and Mental Health*, Methuen, London.
Whiteley, J. S. and Gordon, J. (1979) *Group Approaches in Psychiatry*, Routledge & Kegan Paul, London.

Autobiographical accounts of mental illness

National Schizophrenia Fellowship (1974) *Living with Schizophrenia – By the Relatives*, National Schizophrenia Fellowship, Surbiton.
Reed, D. (1976) *Anna*, Secker & Warburg, London (Penguin edn 1977).
Sutherland, S. (1976) *Breakdown*, Weidenfeld & Nicolson, London.
Wing, J. K. (ed.) (1975) *Schizophrenia from Within*, National Schizophrenia Fellowship, Surbiton.

Appendix B: Glossary

Some common psychiatric terms

acting out (psychoanalytic) unconscious reproduction of conflicts in action rather than words; often applied (imprecisely) to any aggressive or anti-social behaviour

acute of sudden onset and lasting only a short time

adaptive appropriate, meeting the demands of the environment

addiction compulsive craving which the person cannot overcome

aetiology causes

affect [stress on first syllable] mood

affect, flattening of lack of emotional response

affective disorder disorder with mood disturbance as the main feature, e.g. depression, mania

affective lability tendency to rapid mood swings

amnesia loss of memory

amphetamines drug used as stimulant in depression, and as a diet pill in obesity

aphasia (dysphasia) disorder in the use of speech symbols

arteriosclerotic dementia dementia due to damage to the brain following multiple blood clots appearing throughout the brain

assertive training behavioural technique in which client learns to overcome social anxiety by learning to assert himself

ataxia loss of co-ordination of voluntary movements

barbiturates a class of drugs that act as central nervous system depressants

behaviour modification/therapy methods for changing behaviour derived from learning theories

benzodiazepines group of sedative drugs (tranquillisers), e.g. Valium

catatonic type of schizophrenia characterised by psychiatric symptoms such as stupor, holding a bizarre posture for long periods or hyperactivity

catharsis discharge of repressed feelings

central nervous system the brain and the spinal cord

chlorpromazine a major tranquilliser

chorea disorder with jerky, spasmodic movements

chronic lasting for a long time (opposite of 'acute')

cognitive   related to thoughts and ideas

compulsion   feeling of subjective obligation to perform some action, combined with feeling of resistance

conditioning, classical (pavlovian, respondent)   procedure of presenting two stimuli together, the unconditioned stimulus and a neutral (conditioned) stimulus, which causes the subject to respond to the neutral stimulus as to the unconditioned stimulus

conditioning, operant (instrumental)   procedure of following a response by consequences (positive or negative reinforcement or punishment) leading to an increase or decrease in the frequency of the response

confabulation   fabrication to fill in gaps caused by memory loss

cyclothymic   having pronounced mood swings

delirium   acute mental confusion, often with illusions, hallucinations, disorientation

delirium tremens   acute psychosis in alcoholics; main features: clouded consciousness, disorientation, fear, illusions, delusions, hallucinations, restlessness, and tremor

delusion   false belief not held by others of the same social or cultural group

dementia   loss of intellectual faculties

depersonalisation   loss of feeling of being real

desensitisation   a behavioural method used to extinguish phobias; the patient is relaxed, and then gradually exposed to the feared stimulus

disorientation   loss of perception of time and place

dissociation   state in which feelings, thoughts and actions are not in harmony

double bind hypothesis   theory concerning development of schizophrenia: the child is given contradictory messages on different levels and cannot escape or point out the contradiction

dynamic   concerned with cause and effect or drives and motives

empathy   ability to perceive the feelings of another person

endogenous   arising from within

epidemiology   study of the incidence of disease in a population (i.e. the rate at which *new cases* occur over a stated time period) and of the *prevalence* (the absolute number of cases at a particular point of time or over a stated period)

exhibitionism   impulse to exhibit the genitals

flight of ideas   rapid flow of speech characterised by jumping from one topic to another

florid (of symptoms)   dramatic, strikingly obvious

folie a deux   delusional system or other form of psychosis in two individuals

fugue   period of amnesia in which a person may leave home

hallucination   perception that has no basis in reality; can be auditory, visual, gustatory (taste), olfactory (smell), or tactile (feeling)

hebephrenic   type of schizophrenia, often beginning in the teenage years; key features include shallow, inappropriate mood, and giggling

hypnotic   sedative drug prescribed as a sleeping tablet

hypochondriasis   preoccupation with health

hysteria   disorder in which disturbance of consciousness or motor or sensory function seems to procure some psychological advantage

hysterical conversion   unconscious process whereby internal conflict and distress is converted into external, visible disability

ideas of reference   beliefs that everyday events have a special meaning for the individual

illusion   distorted perception

imipramine   drug prescribed for depression

insight   awareness of state of one's mental health

involutional   occurring in middle age

learning theories   theories of behaviour concerned with the relationship between behaviour and its antecedents and consequences

libido   sexual desire

lithium   a mood-stabilising drug

manic   characterised by overactivity and overoptimism, aggressiveness, grandiose ideas

mental disorder   global term referring to all categories of mental disability

morbidity   extent to which a disease is present in a defined population

neuroses   group of mental disorders differentiated from psychoses by such features as insight and milder disturbance

obsession   persistently recurring thought

paraphrenia   paranoid psychosis with hallucinations but few other psychotic symptoms

paranoia   delusions of persecution

parkinsonism   syndrome characterised by tremor, rigidity, mask-like face and loss of spontaneous movement

parnate   an antidepressant drug

personality disorder   disorder distinguished from mental illness as a character type rather than a break in functioning

phenothiazine   tranquillising drug used in treatment of major psychoses

phobia   irrational fear of any object or situation

presenile dementia   dementia occurring before the age of 65

prognosis   forecast of future course or outcome of disorder

prophylaxis   prevention of disorder

psychodrama   form of psychotherapy in which the client enacts important situations in the presence of others, who help him to gain insight into his difficulties

psychogenic   having a psychological cause

psychosis   severe mental illness differentiated from neurosis by such symptoms as lack of insight, delusions, hallucinations and disordered speech

psychosomatic   of physical illness with psychological causes

psychotropic drugs   drugs that affect the mind: antidepressants, major tranquillisers, minor tranquillisers, sedatives and stimulants

puerperal   following childbirth

reactive   provoked by stress

retardation   slowness in speech or actions

schizoaffective   having features of both schizophrenic and manic or depressive illness

simple schizophrenia   type of schizophrenia which develops insidiously and is less obviously psychotic than other types

stupor   state of immobility and lack of response in which consciousness is not entirely lost

syndrome   cluster of symptoms and signs in a familiar pattern

therapeutic community   hospital or other setting which stresses democratic procedures, role-blurring, and making use of the whole community and its everyday incidents as both a context and a means of therapy

thought blocking   breaking off speech, believed to be due to another thought interfering with the original one

thought disorder (formal thought disorder)   abnormality of verbal expression, e.g. blocking, flight of ideas

Some common terms used in research

baseline   record of behaviour made before treatment begins

control, experimental   the control of all extraneous variables (e.g., age, degree of illness) so that any change in the dependent variable (e.g., improvement) can be considered a function of the independent (experimental) variable (e.g., treatment method)

control group   a group equivalent to experimental group in all respects, except for the independent variable, which the experimental group gets and the control group does not

correlation   the degree to which two variables vary together

empirical   based on systematically observed facts and experiments

experimental group   subjects in an experiment who are exposed to the independent or experimental variable (e.g., treatment method), and are matched with the control group in every way except exposure to the experimental variable

hypothesis   a tentative statement to be proved or disproved by evidence

random sample   cases drawn from a population in such a way that all cases in the population have an equal chance of being selected

significant difference   difference (between two samples) so great as to be unlikely to have been caused by chance

Bibliography

Altrocchi, J. (1980) *Abnormal Behavior*, Harcourt Brace Jovanovich, New York.

American Psychiatric Association (1978) *Electroconvulsive Therapy*, Task Force Report, 14, American Psychiatric Association, Washington, September.

Anderson, E. W. and Trethowan, W.H. (1973) *Psychiatry*, 3rd edn, Baillière Tindall, London.

Anstee, B. H. (1978) 'An Alternative to Group Homes,' *British Journal of Psychiatry*, 132, 356–60.

Anthony, E. S. (1969) 'A Clinical Evaluation of Children with Psychotic Parents', *American Journal of Psychiatry*, 126, 177–80.

Apte, R. Z. (1968) *Halfway Houses*, Occasional Papers on Social Administration, No. 27, Bell, London.

Argyle, M., Bryant, B. and Trower, P. (1974) 'Social Skills Training and Psychotherapy: a Comparative Study', *Psychological Medicine*, 4, 435.

Arie, T. (1979) 'A Positive Approach to the Care of Old People with Mental Disorders', in Meacher, Mollie (ed.), *New Methods of Mental Health Care*, Pergamon, Oxford.

Arieti, S. and Bemporad, J. (1980) *Severe and Mild Depression: The Psychotherapeutic Approach*, Tavistock, London.

Atkinson, J. M. (1977) 'Indications for Family Involvement in a Home-based Behavioural Programme with Chronic Schizophrenic Patients', paper delivered at the Annual Conference of the British Association for Behavioural Psychotherapy, Keele University.

Ayllon, T. and Azrin, N. H. (1968) *The Token Economy*, Appleton-Century-Crofts, New York.

Azrin, N. H. (1976) 'Improvements in the Community Reinforcement Approach to Alcoholism', *Behaviour Research and Therapy*, 5, 339–48.

Azrin, N. H., Flores, T. and Kaplan, S. J. (1975) 'Job Finding Club: A Group-assisted Programme for Obtaining Employment', *Behaviour Research and Therapy*, 13, 17–27.

Baldwin, J. (1977) 'Epidemiology of Child Abuse', in Graham, P. J. (ed.), *Epidemiological Approaches in Child Psychiatry*, Academic Press, London.

Barter, J. (1979) 'The Role of the Voluntary Sector in the Provision of

Accommodation and Other Facilities for Mentally Ill and Mentally Handicapped People', in Olsen, M. R. (ed.), *The Care of the Mentally Disordered: An Examination of Some Alternatives to Hospital Care*, BASW, Birmingham.

Bateson, G., Jackson, D., Haley, J. and Weakland, J. (1956) 'Towards a Theory of Schizophrenia', *Behavioral Science*, 1, 251–64.

Baumrind, D. (1967) 'Child Care Practices Anteceding Three Patterns of Pre-school Behaviour', *Genetic Psychology Monographs*, 75, 43–88.

Beck, A. T. (1974) 'Depressive Neurosis', in Arieti, S. (ed.), *American Handbook of Psychiatry*, 2nd edn, Basic Books, New York.

Bednar, R. L. and Lawlis, G. F. (1971) 'Empirical Research in Group Psychotherapy', in Bergin, A. E. and Garfield, S. L. (eds), *Handbook of Psychotherapy and Behavior Change*, Wiley, New York.

Bellack, A. S. and Hersen, M. (eds), (1979) *Research and Practice in Social Skills Training*, Plenum, New York.

Bennett, G. (1970) 'Behavioural Intervention to Prevent Eviction', *Social Work Today*, 1, 11.

Bennun, I. (1980) 'Obsessional Slowness: a Replication and Extension', *Behavior Research and Therapy*, 18, 595–98.

Berkowitz, R., Kuipers, E. and Leff, J. (1981) 'Keeping the Patient Well: Drug and Social Treatments of Schizophrenic Patients', unpublished report, MRC Social Psychiatry Unit, Institute of Psychiatry, London.

Bhanji, S. and Thompson, J. (1974) 'Operant Conditioning in the Treatment of Anorexia Nervosa: A Review and Retrospective Study of 11 Cases', *British Journal of Psychiatry*, 123, 513–18.

Blake, R. and Millard, D. W. (1979) *The Therapeutic Community in Day Care*, Association of Therapeutic Communities.

Bloch, S. (1979) 'Assessment of Patients for Psychotherapy', *British Journal of Psychiatry*, 135, 193–208.

Boudin, H. M. (1972) 'Contingency Contracting as a Therapeutic Tool in the Deceleration of Amphetamine Use', *Behavior Therapy*, 3, 604–8.

Bowlby, J. (1951) *Maternal Care and Mental Health*, World Health Organisation, Geneva.

Braginsky, B. M., Braginsky, D. D. and Ring, K. (1969) *Methods of Madness: the Mental Hospital as a Last Resort*, Holt, Rinehart & Winston, New York.

British Association of Social Workers (Mental Health Section) (1974) 'Report of the Discussion Within the Working Party about the Role of the Social Worker and Social Services in the Care of the Mentally Ill', in *Aspects of the Social Care of the Mentally Ill: A Discussion Paper*, BASW, Birmingham.

Brown, G. W. and Birley, J. L. T. (1968) 'Crises and Life Changes and the Onset of Schizophrenia', *Journal of Health and Social Behaviour*, 9, 203–14.

Brown, G. W. and Birley, J. L. T. (1970) 'Social Precipitants of Severe Psychiatric Disorders', in Hare, E. H. and Wing, J. K. (eds), *Psychiatric Epidemiology*, Oxford University Press for Nuffield Provincial Hospitals Trust, Oxford.

Brown, G. W., Birley, J. L. T., and Wing, J. K. (1972) 'Influence of Family Life on the Course of Schizophrenic Disorders: a Replication', *British Journal of Psychiatry*, 121, 241–58.

Brown, G. W., Bone, M., Dalison, B. and Wing, J. K. (1966) *Schizophrenia and Social Care*, Oxford University Press, Oxford.

Brown, G. W. and Harris, T. (1978) *The Social Origins of Depression*, Tavistock, London.

Brown, G. W., Sklair, F., Harris, T. O. and Birley, J. L. T. (1973) 'Life Events and Psychiatric Disorders Part II: Nature of Causal Link', *Psychological Medicine*, 3, 159–76.

Canever, N. (1980) personal communication by letter.

Caplan, G. (1964) *Principles of Preventive Psychiatry*, Tavistock, London.

Carstairs, G. M., O'Connor, N. and Rawnsley, K. (1956) 'Organization of a Hospital Workshop for Chronic Psychotic Patients', *British Journal of Preventive and Social Medicine*, 10, 136–40.

Catts, S. and McConaghy, N. (1975) 'Ritual Prevention in the Treatment of Obsessive Compulsive Neurosis', *Australia and New Zealand Journal of Psychiatry*, 9, 37–41.

Cautela, J. R. (1970) 'The Treatment of Alcoholism by Covert Sensitization', *Psychotherapy*, 7, 86–90.

Cheek, F. E., Laucius, J., Mahncke, M. and Beck, R. (1971a) 'A Behavior Modification Training Program for Parents of Convalescent Schizophrenics', in Rubin, R., Fensterheim, H., Lazarus, A. and Franks, C. (eds), *Advances in Behavior Therapy*, Academic Press, New York.

Cheek, F. E., Franks, C. M., Laucius, S. and Burtle, W. (1971b) 'Behavior Modification Training for Wives of Alcoholics', *Quarterly Journal of Studies in Alcohol*, 32, 456–61.

Chiles, J. A., Stauss, F. S. and Benjamin, L. S. (1980) 'Marital Conflict and Sexual Dysfunction in Alcoholic and Non-alcoholic Couples', *British Journal of Psychiatry*, 137, 266–73.

Clare, A. (1976) *Psychiatry in Dissent*, Tavistock, London.

Clare, A. (1979) 'Ethics in Psychiatry', in Gaind, R. and Hudson, B. L. (eds), *Current Themes in Psychiatry II*, Macmillan, London.

Clare, A. (1980) 'Current Trends in the Treatment of Depression', in Tennant, T. G. (ed.), *Current Trends in Treatment in Psychiatry*, Pitman, London.

Clarke, A. M. and Clarke, A. D. B. (1976) *Early Experience: Myth and Evidence*, Open Books, London.

Clarke, J. (1971) 'An Analysis of Crisis Management by Mental Welfare Officers', *British Journal of Social Work*, 1, 27–39.

Cooper, B., Harwin, B. G., Depla, C. and Shepherd, M. (1975) 'Mental Health Care in the Community: an Evaluative Study', *Psychological Medicine*, 5, 4, 372–80.

Cooper, P. (1979) 'Employment Problems and Prospects for Chronic Patients', in Meacher, M. (ed.), *New Methods of Mental Health Care*, Pergamon, Oxford.

Cooper, S. F., Leach, C., Storer, D. and Tonge, W. L. (1977) 'The Children of Psychiatric Patients: Clinical Findings', *British Journal of Psychiatry*,

131, 514–22.

Craft, M. (1966) *Psychopathic Disorders*, Pergamon, Oxford.

Creer, C. and Wing, J. K. (1974) *Schizophrenia at Home*, National Schizophrenia Fellowship, Surbiton.

Crow, T. J. (1979) Editorial, 'The Scientific Status of Electro-convulsive Therapy', *Psychological Medicine*, 9, 401–8.

Crowe, M. J. (1978) 'Behavioural Approaches to Marital and Family Therapy', in Gaind, R. and Hudson, B. L. (eds), *Current Themes in Psychiatry I*, Macmillan, London.

Cumming, J. and Cumming, E. (1957) 'Social Equilibrium and Social Change in the Large Mental Hospital', in Greenblatt, M. (ed.), *The Patient and the Mental Hospital*, The Free Press, New York, pp. 49–72.

Custance, J. (1952) 'The Universe of Bliss and the Universe of Horror: A Description of a Manic-Depressive Psychosis', in Custance, J. (ed.), *Wisdom Madness and Folly*, reprinted in Kaplan, B. (ed.), *The Inner World of Mental Illness* (1964), Harper & Row, New York.

Dawson, H. (1972) 'Reasons for Compulsory Admission', in Wing, J. K. and Hailey, A. (eds), *Evaluating a Community Psychiatric Service*, Oxford University Press, Oxford.

Decker, B. J. and Stubblebine, J. M. (1972) 'Crisis Intervention and the Prevention of Chronic Disability', *American Journal of Psychiatry*, 129, 6.

DeRisi, W. J., Myron, M. and Goding, M. (1976) 'A Workshop to Train Community-care Staff to Use Behavior Modification Techniques', *Hospital and Community Psychiatry*, 26, 636–7.

Dohrenwend, B. S. and Dohrenwend, B. P. (eds) (1974) *Stressful Life Events: Their Nature and Effects*, Wiley, New York.

Dunham, H. W. (1965) *Community and Schizophrenia*, Wayne State University Press, Detroit.

Eisenberg, L. (1977) 'Psychiatry and Society', *New England Journal of Medicine*, 21 April 1977.

Emrick, C. D. (1975) 'Review of Psychologically Orientated Treatments of Alcoholism', *Journal of Studies in Alcoholism*, 36(1), 88.

Engel, G. (1961) 'Is Grief a Disease?', *Psychosomatic Medicine*, 23.

Ewing, C. P. (1978) *Crisis Intervention as Psychotherapy*, Oxford University Press, New York.

Eysenck, H. J. (1970) *Crime and Personality*, Granada Press, St Albans.

Fairweather, G. W., Sanders, D. M., Maynard, H. and Cressler, D. L. (1969) *Community Care for the Mentally Ill*, Aldine, Chicago.

Falloon, I., Lindley, P., McDonald, R. and Marks, I. M. (1977) 'Social Skills Training of Out-Patient Groups: A Controlled Study of Rehearsal and Homework', *British Journal of Psychiatry*, 131, 599–609.

Fernandez, J. (1982) 'The Token Economy', in Gaind, R. and Hudson, B. L. (eds), *Current Themes in Psychiatry III*, Macmillan, London.

Fischer, J. (1978) *Effective Casework Practice*, McGraw-Hill, New York.

Fitzgerald, R. (1982) 'Sociological Perspectives on Mental Health and Illness', in Gaind, R. and Hudson, B. L. (eds), *Current Themes in Psychiatry III*, Macmillan, London.

Flomenhaft, K. and Langsley, D. G. (1971) 'After Crisis', *Mental Hygiene*, 5, 4, 473–7.

Flowers, J. V. (1975) 'Simulation and Role Playing Methods', in Kanfer, F. H. and Goldstein, A. P. (eds), *Helping People Change*, Pergamon, New York.

Fox, R. (1973) 'The Management of the Suicidal Patient: A Psychiatrist's View', in Varah, C. (ed.), *The Samaritans in the Seventies*, Constable, London.

Freeman, H. (1978) 'Mental Health and the Environment', *British Journal of Psychiatry*, 132, 113–24.

Freeman, H. E. and Simmons, O. G. (1958) 'Mental Patients in the Community: Family Settings and Performance Levels', *American Sociological Review*, 23, 2.

Friedman, A. S. (1975) 'Interaction of Drug Therapy with Marital Therapy in Depressive Patients', *Archives of General Psychiatry*, 32, 619–37.

Fry, A. (1978) 'Some Aspects of the Problem Orientated Medical Record in General Psychiatry', in Gaind, R. and Hudson, B. L. (eds), *Current Themes in Psychiatry I*, Macmillan, London.

Galle, O. Gove, W. R. and McPherson, J. M. (1972) 'Population Density Pathology', *Science*, 176, 23–30.

Gambrill, E. (1977) *Behavior Modification*, Jossey-Bass, San Francisco and London.

Garfield, E. (1979) 'Electroconvulsive Therapy: Malignant or Maligned?', *Current Comments*, 42, 15 October.

Garmezy, N. (1974) 'Children at Risk: the Search for the Antecedents of Schizophrenia Part II: Ongoing Research Programs, Issues and Intervention', *Schizophrenia Bulletin*, 9, 55–125.

Gattoni, F. and Tarnopolsky, A. (1973) 'Aircraft Noise and Psychiatric Morbidity', *Psychological Medicine*, 3, 516–20.

Gibbons, J. S., Butler, J., Urwin, P. and Gibbons, J. L. (1978) 'Evaluation of a Social Work Service for Self-poisoning Patients', *British Journal of Psychiatry*, 133, 111–18.

Gleisner, J., Hewett, S. and Mann, S. (1972) 'Reasons for Admission to Hospital', in Wing, J. K. and Hailey, A. M. (eds), *Evaluating a Community Psychiatric Service*, Oxford University Press, Oxford.

Goffman, E. (1961) *Asylums*, Archer Books, Doubleday, New York.

Goldberg, D. and Huxley, P. (1980) *Mental Illness in the Community*, Tavistock, London.

Goldberg, E. M. and Warburton, R. W. (1979) *Ends and Means in Social Work*, National Institute for Social Work, Social Services Library No. 35, Allen & Unwin, London.

Goldberg, E. M., Williams, B. T. and Mortimer, A. (1970) *Helping the Aged*, Allen & Unwin, London.

Goldstein, A. P. and Simonson, N. R. (1971) 'Social Psychological Approaches to Psychotherapy Research', in Bergin, A. E. and Garfield, S. (eds), *Handbook of Psychotherapy and Behavior Change*, Wiley, New York.

Goldstein, R. S. and Baer, D. M. (1976) 'RSVP: A Procedure to Increase the Personal Mail and Number of Correspondents for Nursing Home Residents', *Behavior Therapy*, 7, 348–54.

Gordon, M. (1978) 'Observations on Statutory Examinations', *Social Work Today*, 9, 42, 24–5.

Gostin, L. (1975) *The Mental Health Act from 1959 to 1975. Observations, Analysis, and Proposals for Reform*, MIND (National Association for Mental Health), London.

Gove, W. R., Hughes, M. and Galle, O. M. (1978) 'Overcrowding in the Home: An Empirical Investigation of its possible Pathological Consequences', *American Sociological Review*, 44, February.

Grad, J. and Sainsbury, P. (1968) 'The Effects that Patients have on their Families in a Community Care and a Control Psychiatric Service', *British Journal of Psychiatry*, 114, 265.

Gray, B. and Isaacs, B. (1979) *Care of the Elderly Mentally Infirm*, Tavistock, London.

Greene, J. G., Nicol, R. and Jamieson, H. (1979) 'Reality Orientation with Psychogeriatric Patients', *Behaviour Research and Therapy*, 17, 618–21.

Gunderson, J. G., Autry, J. H. III, Mosher, L. R. and Buchsbaum, S. (1974) 'Special Report: Schizophrenia, 1974', *Schizophrenia Bulletin*, 9, 16–54.

Gunn, J. (1978) 'The Treatment of Psychopaths', in Gaind, R. and Hudson, B. L. (eds), *Current Themes in Psychiatry I*, Macmillan, London.

Gunn, J. and Robertson, G. (1976) 'Psychopathic Personality: a Conceptual Problem', *Psychological Medicine*, 6, 631–4.

Gunn, J., Robertson, G., Dell, S. and Way, C. (1978) *Psychiatric Aspects of Imprisonment*, Academic Press, London.

Hare. E. M. and Shaw, G. K. (1965) *Mental Health on a New Housing Estate*, Oxford University Press, Oxford.

Hare, R. D. and Schalling, D. (1978) *Psychopathy: Theory and Research*, Wiley, London.

Harwin, J. (1979) 'Recognition of Alcohol Problems', *Social Work Today*, 10, 41, 11–12.

Henderson, A. S. (1977) 'The Social Network, Support and Neurosis', *British Journal of Psychiatry*, 131, 185–91.

Henderson, J. D. and Scoles, P. E. (1970) 'A Community-based Behavioral Operant Environment for Psychotic Men', *Behavior Therapy*, 1, 245–51.

Hetherington, E. M. and Martin, B. (1972) 'Family Interaction and Psychopathology in Children', in Quay, H. C. and Werry, J. S. (eds), *Psychopathological Disorders of Childhood*, Wiley, New York.

Hewett, S. (1979) 'Somewhere to Live: a Pilot Study of Hostel Care', in Olsen, M. R. (ed.), *The Care of the Mentally Disordered: an Examination of some Alternatives to Hospital Care*, BASW, Birmingham.

Hill, J. M. (1978) 'The Psychological Impact of Unemployment', *New Society*, 19 January 1978.

Hirsch, S. R., Gaind, R., Rohde, P. D., Stevens, B. C. and Wing, J. K. (1973) 'Out-patient Maintenance of Chronic Schizophrenic Patients with Long-acting Fluphenazine: Double-blind Placebo Trial', *British Medical Journal*, 1, 633–7.

Hirsch, S. R. and Leff, J. P. (1975) *Abnormalities in Parents of Schizophrenics: a Review of the Literature and an Investigation of Communication Aspects and Deviances*, Oxford University Press, Oxford.

Hirsch, S. R., Platt, P., Weyman, A. and Knights, A. (1979) 'A Brief Hospitalisation Policy: the Effects upon Patients and their Families', in Meacher, M. (ed.), *New Methods of Mental Health Care*, Pergamon, Oxford.

Hoenig, J. and Hamilton, M. W. (1969) *The De-segregation of the Mentally Ill*, Routledge & Kegan Paul, London.

Hudson, B. L. (1975a) 'A Behavior Modification Project with Chronic Schizophrenics in the Community', *Behavior Research and Therapy*, 13, 239–41.

Hudson, B. L. (1975b) 'An Inadequate Personality', *Social Work Today*, 6, 506.

Hudson, B.L. (1976) 'The Haunted Bedroom', *Social Work Today*, 8, 10.

Hughes, D. (1978) *How Psychiatric Patients Manage Out of Hospital: Community Provision, Living Standards and Financial Needs*, The Disability Alliance, London.

Hunt, G. M. and Azrin, N. H. (1973) 'A Community Reinforcement Approach to Alcoholism', *Behaviour Research and Therapy*, 2, 91–104.

Hunt, M. (1979) 'Possibilities and Problems of Inter-disciplinary Teamwork', in Marshall, M., Preston-Shoot, M. and Wincot, E. (eds), *Teamwork: For and Against*, BASW, Birmingham.

Iversen, L. L. (1978) 'The Dopamine Hypothesis', in Wing, J. K. (ed.), *Schizophrenia: Towards a New Synthesis*, Academic Press, London.

Jayaratne, S. and Levy, R. L. (1979) *Empirical Clinical Practice*, Columbia University Press, New York.

Jehu, D. (1979) *Sexual Dysfunction*, Wiley, Chichester.

Jenkins, J., Felce, D , Lunt, B. and Powell, L. (1977) 'Increasing Activity in Old People's Homes by Providing Recreational Materials', *Behaviour Research and Therapy*, 15, 429–34.

Johnson, F. N. (1974a) 'Lithium Therapy and Its Implications', *Social Work Today*, 5, 6.

Johnson, F. N. (1974b) 'Lithium Therapy and the Psychiatric Social Worker', *Social Work Today*, 5, 11.

Johnstone, E., Deakin, J. F. W., Lawler, P., Frith, C. D., Stevens, M., McPherson, K. and Crow, T. J. (1980) 'The Northwick Park ECT Trial', *Lancet*, 2, 1317–20.

Kendell, R. E. (1974) 'A New Look at Hysteria', *Medicine*, 30, 1780–83.

Kolvin, I., Garside, R. F., Nicol, A. R., Macmillian, A., Wolstenholme, F. and Leitch, I. M. (1977) 'Familial and Sociological Correlates of Behavioural and Sociometric Deviance in 8-year-old Children', in Graham, P. J. (ed.), *Epidemiological Approaches in Child Psychiatry*, Academic Press, London.

Kornhauser, A. (1965) *Mental Health of the Industrial Worker*, Wiley, New York.

Kreitman, N., Collins, J., Nelson, B. and Troop, J. (1970) 'Neurosis and

Marital Interaction', *British Journal of Psychiatry*, 117, 33–58.

Kreitman, N., Collins, J., Nelson, B. and Troop, J. (1971) 'Neuroses and Marital Interaction', *British Journal of Psychiatry*, 119, 223–52.

Kutner, L. (1962) 'The Illusion of Due Process in Commitment Proceedings', *Northwestern University Law Review*, 57, 383–99.

Lader, M. (1978) 'Some Psychophysiological Aspects of Anxiety', in Gaind, R. and Hudson, B. L. (eds), *Current Themes in Psychiatry I*, Macmillan, London.

Laing, R. D. and Esterson, D. (1964) *Sanity, Madness and the Family*, Tavistock, London.

Langsley, D. G. and Kaplan, D. (1968) *The Treatment of Families in Crisis*, Grune & Stratton, New York.

Langsley, D. G., Flomenhaft, K. and Machotka, P. (1969) 'Follow-up Evaluation of Family Crisis Therapy', *American Journal of Orthopsychiatry*, 39, 753.

Langsley, D. R., Machotka, P. and Flomenhaft, K. (1971) 'Avoiding Mental Hospital Admission: A Follow Up Study', *American Journal of Psychiatry*, 127, 1391–4.

Lavan, A. (1980) 'Putting it on Record', *Community Care*, 19 June.

Leff, J. P. (1978) 'Social and Psychological Causes of the Acute Attack', in Wing, J. K. (ed.), *Schizophrenia: Towards a New Synthesis*, Academic Press, London.

Leff, J. P. and Wing, J. K. (1971) 'Trial of Maintenance Therapy in Schizophrenia', *British Medical Journal*, 3, 599–604.

Leonard, W. (1927) *The Locomotive God*, Appleton-Century-Crofts, New York.

Lewinsohn, P. M. (1974) 'A Behavioral Approach to Depression', in Friedman, R. J. and Katz, M. M. (eds), *The Psychology of Depression*, V. H. Winston, Washington, D. C.

Liberman, R. P. and Bryan, E. (1977) 'Behavior Therapy in a Community Mental Health Center', *American Journal of Psychiatry*, 134, 4, 401–6

Liberman, R. P., King, L. W., DeRisi, W. J. and McCann, M. (1975) *Personal Effectiveness*, Research Press, Champaign, Ill.

Liberman, R. P. and Raskin, D. E. (1971) 'Depression: a Behavioural Formulation', *Archives of General Psychiatry*, 24, 515–23.

Lidz, T., Cornelison, A. R. and Fleck, S. (1965) *Schizophrenia and the Family*, International Universities Press, New York.

Lindemann, E. (1944) 'Symptomatology and Management of Acute Grief', *American Journal of Psychiatry*, 101, 141–8.

Linford-Rees, W. L. (1976) *A Short Textbook of Psychiatry*, 2nd edn, Hodder & Stoughton, London.

Linsk, N., Howe, M. W. and Pinkston, E. M. (1975) 'Behavioral Group Work in a Home for the Aged', *Social Work*, 20, 454–63.

Lloyd, B. (1971) 'A Relatives Group', Unpublished paper circulated by the Orpington Mental Health Association, Anchor House, Station Road, Orpington, Kent.

Lund, C. A. and Gardiner, A. Q. (1977) 'The Gaslight Phenomenon – An Institutional Variant', *British Journal of Psychiatry*, 131, 533–4.

McAuley, R. R. (1980) 'Commentary on "Current Trends in the Treatment of Depression"', in Tennant, T. G. (ed.), *Current Trends in Treatment in Psychiatry*, Pitman, London.

McAuley, R. and McAuley, P. (1977) *Child Behaviour Problems*, Macmillan, London.

McAuley, R. and McAuley, P. (1980) 'The Effectiveness of Behaviour Modification with Families', *British Journal of Social Work*, 10, 43–54.

McAuley, R. R. and Quinn, J. T. (1971) 'Behavioural Analysis, Treatment and Theoretical Implications of a Case of Depression', Paper presented at the Third Annual Conference of the Behavioural Engineering Association, Wexford, Ireland.

McClannahan, L. E. and Risley, T. R. (1975) 'Design of Living Environments for Nursing Home Residents: Increasing Participation in Recreational Activities', *Journal of Applied Behavior Analysis*, 8, 261–8.

McKnew, D. H., Cytryn, L., Efron, A. M., Gershon, E. S. and Bunney, W. E. (1979) 'Offspring of Patients with Affective Disorders', *British Journal Psychiatry*, 134, 148–52.

Mantus, L. (1973) 'An Illness Like Any Other', *New Society*, 19 April, 131–2.

Marks, I. M. (1969) *Fears and Phobias*, Heinemann, London.

Marks, I. M. (1973) 'Research in Neurosis: A Selective Review 1: Causes and Courses', *Psychological Medicine*, 3, 436–53.

Marks, I. M. (1974) 'Research in Neurosis: A Selective Review 2: Treatment', *Psychological Medicine*, 4, 1, 89–109.

Marks, I. M. (1978) 'Behavioral Psychotherapy of Neurotic Disorders', in Garfield, S. and Bergin, A. E. (eds), *Handbook of Psychotherapy and Behavior Change* (2nd edn) Wiley, New York.

Martindale, B. and Bottomley, V. (1980) 'The Management of Families with Huntington's Chorea', *Journal of Child Psychology and Psychiatry*, 21, 4, 343–51.

Marzillier, J. (1978) 'Outcome Studies of Skills Training', in Trower, P., Bryant, B. and Argyle, M. (eds), *Social Skills and Mental Health*, Methuen, London.

Masters, W. H. and Johnson, V. E. (1970) *Human Sexual Inadequacy*, Little, Brown & Co., Boston.

Mathews, A. M., Teasdale, J., Munby, M., Johnston, D. W. and Shaw, P. M. (1977) 'A Home Based Treatment Programme for Agoraphobia', *Behavior Therapy*, 8, 915–24.

Mathews, R. M., Whang, P. L. and Fawcett, S. B. (1980) 'Development and Validation of an Occupational Skills Assessment Instrument', *Behavioral Assessment*, 2, 71–85.

Mayer, J. E. and Timms, N. (1970) *The Client Speaks*, Routledge & Kegan Paul, London.

Meacher, Michael (1971) *Scrounging on the Welfare*, Arrow, London.

Meichenbaum, D. (1977) *Cognitive Behavior Modification*, Plenum, New York.

Mendelsohn, M. (1974) *Psychoanalytic Concepts of Depression*, Spectrum Publications, Flushing, New York.

Meyer, M.-L. (1978) *Counselling Families of Alcoholics*, London Council on Alcoholism.

Miles, A. (1977) 'Staff Relations in Psychiatric Hospitals', *British Journal of Psychiatry*, 130, 84–8.

Millard, D. W. (1981a) personal communication by letter.

Millard, D. W. (1981b) 'The Therapeutic Community in the Seventies', in Gaind, R. and Hudson, B. L. (eds), *Current Themes in Psychiatry III*, Macmillan, London.

MIND (1975) *Starting and Running a Group Home*, MIND (National Association for Mental Health), London.

MIND (1978) *Nobody Wants You: 40 Cases of Discrimination at Work*, MIND (National Association for Mental Health), London.

MIND (1979) *Your Money in Hospital*, MIND (National Association for Mental Health), London.

Mishler, E. G. and Waxler, H. E. (1963) 'Decision Process in Psychiatric Hospitalisation: Patients Referred, Accepted and Admitted to Psychiatric Hospital', *American Sociological Review*, 28, 576.

Monahan, J. (1975) 'The Prediction of Violence', in Chappell, D. and Monahan, J. (eds), *Violence and Criminal Justice*, Lexington Books (D. C. Heath), Lexington, Mass.

Moore, N. C. (1974) 'Psychiatric Illness and Living in Flats', *British Journal of Psychiatry*, 125, 500–7.

Morgan, H. G. (1979) 'The Self-poisoning Patient. Treatment and Prevention', in Gaind, R. and Hudson, B. L. (eds), *Current Themes in Psychiatry II*, Macmillan, London.

Murray, J. (1977) *Better Prospects: Rehabilitation in Mental Illness Hospitals*, MIND (National Association for Mental Health), London.

National Schizophrenia Fellowship (1974a) *Living with Schizophrenia: by the Relatives*, National Schizophrenia Fellowship, Surbiton.

National Schizophrenia Fellowship (1974b) *Social Provision for Sufferers from Chronic Schizophrenia*, National Schizophrenia Fellowship, Surbiton.

National Schizophrenia Fellowship (1979) *Home Sweet Nothing*, National Schizophrenia Fellowship, Surbiton.

Newman, N. (1970) 'The Children of Schizophrenics', Thesis submitted for the Diploma in Social and Administrative Studies, University of Oxford.

Newson-Smith, J. G. B. and Hirsch, S. R. (1979) 'A Comparison of Social Workers and Psychiatrists in Evaluating Parasuicide', *British Journal of Psychiatry*, 134, 335–42.

O'Brien, F. and Azrin, N. H. (1973) 'Interaction-priming: a Method of Reinstating Patient-Family Relationships', *Behaviour Research and Therapy*, 11, 133–6.

Office of Health Economics (1979) *Schizophrenia: Biochemical Impairments; Social Handicaps?*, Office of Health Economics, London.

Oliver, J. (1981) 'The Behavioural Treatment of Obsessional House Cleaning in a "Personality Disordered" Client: a Case Study', *International Journal of Behavioural Social Work and Abstracts*, 1, 1, 39–53.

Olsen, M. R. (1976a) 'The Personal and Social Consequences of the Discharge of the Long-Stay Psychiatric Patient from the North Wales

Hospital, Denbigh (1965–66)', Ph.D. thesis, University of Wales.

Olsen, M. R. (1976b) 'Boarding-out the Long-stay Psychiatric Patient', in Olsen, M. R. (ed.), *Differential Approaches in Social Work with the Mentally Disordered*, BASW, Birmingham.

Olsen, M. R. (1979a) 'The Chronic Psychiatric Patient – Techniques to Improve Social Functioning', in Olsen, M. R. (ed.), *The Care of the Mentally Disordered*, BASW, Birmingham.

Olsen, M. R. (1979b) 'A Model of Emergency Management', in Meacher, M. (ed.), *New Methods of Mental Health Care*, Pergamon, Oxford.

Olshansky, S. (1962) 'Chronic Sorrow: A Response to Having a Mentally Defective Child', *Social Casework*, XLIII, April, 190–93.

Orford, J. (1975) 'Alcoholism and Marriage: the Argument Against Specialism', *Quarterly Journal of Studies on Alcohol*, 36, 1537–63.

Ovenstone, I. M. K. (1973) 'The Development of Neurosis in the Wives of Neurotic Men', *British Journal of Psychiatry*, 122, 711–17.

Paolino, T. J. and McCurdy, B. J. (1977) *The Alcoholic Marriage*, Grune & Stratton, New York.

Parad, H. G. (1976) 'Crisis Intervention in Mental Health Emergencies', in Olsen, M. R. (ed.), *Differential Approaches in Social Work with the Mentally Disordered*, BASW, Birmingham.

Patterson, G. R., Cobb, J. A. and Ray, R. S. (1973) 'A Social Engineering Technology for Retraining the Families of Aggressive Boys' in Adams, H. E. and Unikel, J. P. (eds), *Issues and Trends in Behavior Therapy*, Charles C. Thomas, Springfield, Illinois.

Paykel, E. S. (1978) 'Contribution of Life Events to Causation of Psychiatric Illness', *Psychological Medicine*, 8, 245–53.

Paykel, E. S., Myers, J. K., Diendelt, M. N., Klerman, G. L., Lindenthal, J. J. and Pepper, M. P. (1969) 'Life Events and Depression', *Archives of General Psychiatry*, 21, 753–60.

Powell, E., Felce, D., Jenkins, J. and Lunt, B. (1979) 'Increasing Engagement in a Home for the Elderly by Providing an Indoor Gardening Activity', *Behaviour Research and Therapy*, 17, 127–35.

Priest, R. G. and Steinert, J. (1977) *Insanity*, Macdonald & Evans, Plymouth.

Priest, R. G. and Woolfson, G. (1978) *Minski's Handbook of Psychiatry*, Heinemann, London.

Priestley, D. (1979) 'Helping a Self-help Group' (Part II of 'Schizophrenia and the Family'), in Wing, J. K. and Olsen, M. R. (eds), *Community Care for the Mentally Disabled*, Oxford University Press, Oxford.

Prins, H. A. (1975) 'A Danger to Themselves and to Others: Social Workers and Potentially Dangerous Clients', *British Journal of Social Work*, 5, 297–309.

Prins, H. A. (1980) *Offenders: Deviants or Patients?*, Tavistock, London.

Pritlove, J. H. (1976) 'Evaluating a Group Home: Problems and Results', *British Journal of Social Work*, 6, 3, 353–76.

Quay, H. C. (1965) 'Psychopathic Personality as Pathological Stimulation-seeking', *American Journal of Psychiatry*, 122, 180–83.

Rachman, S. (1976) 'The Modification of Obsessions', *Behaviour Research and Therapy*, 14, 437–43.

Ramsay, R. W. (1976) 'A Case Study in Bereavement Therapy', in Eysenck, H. J. (ed.), *Case Studies in Behaviour Therapy*, Routledge & Kegan Paul, London.

Ramsay, R. W. and Happée, J. A. (1977) 'The Stress of Bereavement: Components and Treatment', in Spielberger, C. D. and Sarason, I. G. (eds), *Stress and Anxiety*, vol. 4, Wiley, New York.

Ramsay, S. (1976) 'Huntington's Chorea Comes Out Of Hiding', *Social Work Today*, 8, 8, 12–13.

Raphael, B. (1977) 'Preventive Intervention with the Recently Bereaved', *Archives of General Psychiatry*, 34, 1450–54.

Rapoport, L. (1962) 'The State of Crisis: Some Theoretical Considerations', *The Social Service Review*, 36, reprinted 1965 in Parad, H. J. (ed.), *Crisis Intervention*, Family Service Association of America, New York.

Rapoport, L. (1970) 'Crisis Intervention as a Mode of Brief Treatment', in Roberts, R. W. and Nee, R. H. (eds), *Theories of Social Casework*, University of Chicago Press, Chicago.

Rice, E. P., Ekdahl, M. C. and Miller, L. (1971) *Children of Mentally Ill Parents*, Behavior Publications, New York.

Richman, N. (1977) 'Behaviour Problems in Pre-school Children: Family and Social Factors', *British Journal of Psychiatry*, 131, 523–7.

Rosenhan, D. L. (1973) 'On Being Sane in Insane Places', *Science*, 179, 250–58.

Ross, R. R. and McKay, H. B. (1979) *Self Mutilation*, Lexington Books (D. C. Heath), Lexington, Mass.

Rothaus, P., Hanson, P. G., Cleveland, S. E. and Johnson, D. L. (1963) 'Describing Psychiatric Hospitalization: a Dilemma', *American Psychologist*, 18, 85–9.

Royal College of Psychiatrists (1979) *Alcohol and Alcoholism*, Tavistock, London.

Rush, A. J., Beck, A. T., Kovacs, J. and Hollan, S. (1977) 'Comparative Efficacy of Cognitive Therapy and Pharmacotherapy in the Treatment of Depressed Out-patients', *Cognitive Therapy and Research*, 1, 17–37.

Rutter, M. (1966) *Children of Sick Parents*, Oxford University Press, Oxford.

Rutter, M. L., Cox, A., Tupling, C., Berger, M. and Yule, W. (1976) 'Attainment and Adjustment in Two Geographical Areas 1: The Prevalence of Psychiatric Disorder', *British Journal of Psychiatry*, 126, 493–509.

Rutter, M. and Hersov, L. (1976) *Child Psychiatry: Modern Approaches*, Blackwell, Oxford.

Rutter, M. and Madge, N. (1976) *Cycles of Disadvantage*, Heinemann, London.

Rutter, M., Quinton, D. and Yule, W. (1977) *Family Pathology and Disorder in Childhood*, Wiley, London.

Rutter, M. L., Yule, B., Quinton, D., Rowlands, O., Yule, W. and Berger, M. (1975) 'Attainment and Adjustment in Two Geographical Areas III: Some Factors Accounting for Area Differences', *British Journal of Psychiatry*, 126, 520–33.

Ryan, P. (1979) 'Residential Care for the Mentally Disabled', in Wing, J. K. and Olsen, M. R. (eds), *Community Care for the Mentally Disabled*, Oxford University Press, Oxford.

Ryan, P. and Hewett, S. H. (1976) 'A Pilot Study of Hostels for the Mentally Ill', *Social Work Today*, 6, 774–8.

Ryan, P. and Wing, J. K. (1979) 'Patterns of Residential Care: A Study of Hostels and Group Homes used by four Local Authorities to support Mentally Ill People in the Community', in Olsen, M. R. (ed.), *The Care of the Mentally Disordered: An Examination of Some Alternatives to Hospital Care*, BASW, Birmingham.

Sainsbury, P. (1973) 'Suicide: Opinions and Facts', *Proceedings of the Royal Society of Medicine*, 66, 579.

Sampson, H., Messinger, S. L. and Towne, R. (1965) 'Family Processes and Becoming a Mental Patient', in Zald, M. N. (ed.), *Social Welfare Institutions*, Wiley, New York.

Sanson-Fisher, R. W., Poole, A. D. and Harker, J. (1979) 'Behavioural Analysis of Ward Rounds Within a General Hospital Psychiatric Unit', *Behaviour Research and Therapy*, 17, 333–48.

Saunders, D. (1977) 'Marital Violence: Dimensions of the Problem and Modes of Intervention', *Journal of Marriage and Family Counselling*, January.

Schaffer, J. B. and Tyler, J. D. (1979) 'Degree of Sobriety in Male Alcoholics and Coping Styles used by their Wives', *British Journal of Psychiatry*, 135, 431–7.

Scheff, T. J. (1974) 'The Labeling Theory of Mental Illness', *American Sociological Review*, 39, 444–52.

Schofield, W. (1964) *Psychotherapy, the Purchase of Friendship*, Prentice-Hall, Englewood Cliffs, New Jersey.

Scott, P. D. (1978) 'The Psychiatry of Kidnapping and Hostage-Taking', in Gaind, R. and Hudson, B. L. (eds), *Current Themes in Psychiatry I*, Macmillan, London.

Seebohm Committee (1968) *Report of the Committee on Local Authority and Allied Personal Social Services*, Cmnd 3703 (July 1968), HMSO.

Segal, S. P. and Aviram, U. (1978) *The Mentally Ill in Community-based Sheltered Care*, Wiley, New York.

Seixas, J. (1980) *How to Cope with an Alcoholic Parent*, Canongate, Edinburgh.

Seligman, M. E. P. (1975) *Helplessness*, W. H. Freeman, San Francisco.

Sheldon, B. (1978) 'Theory and Practice in Social Work: A Re-examination of a Tenuous Relationship', *British Journal of Social Work*, 8, 1, 1–22.

Sheppard, M. L. (1960) 'Psychotherapy with a Small Group of Chronic Schizophrenic Patients', *British Journal of Psychiatric Social Work*, 8, 3.

Sims, A. C. P. (1978) 'Prognosis in Severe Neurosis', in Gaind, R. and Hudson, B. L. (eds), *Current Themes in Psychiatry I*, Macmillan, London.

Singer, M. T. and Wynne, L. C. (1965) 'Thought Disorder and Family Relations of Schizophrenics IV: Results and Implications', *Archives of General Psychiatry*, 12, 201–12.

Slater, H. (1979) 'Community Care for the Mentally Frail', in Olsen, M. R. (ed.), *The Care of the Mentally Disordered: An Examination of Some Alternatives to Hospital Care*, BASW, Birmingham.

Smith, G. (1979) 'Family Substitute Care in the Rehabilitation of the Discharged Psychiatric Patient', in Olsen, M. R. (ed.), *The Care of the Mentally Disordered: an Examination of Some Alternatives to Hospital Care*, BASW, Birmingham, 141–8.

Smith, R. J. (1978) *The Psychopath in Society*, Academic Press, New York.

Smith, S. M., Hanson, R. and Noble, S. (1973) 'Parents of Battered Babies: a Controlled Study', *British Medical Journal*, IV, 388–91.

Sobell, L., Sobell, M. and Christelman, W. (1972) 'The Myth of "One Drink"', *Behaviour Research and Therapy*, 10, 119–23.

Sobell, M. B. and Sobell, L. C. (1978) *Behavioral Treatment of Alcohol Problems: Individualized Therapy and Controlled Drinking*, Plenum, New York.

Spratley, T. A. (1978) 'Aspects of the Management of Alcoholism', in Gaind, R. and Hudson, B. L. (eds), *Current Themes in Psychiatry I*, Macmillan, London.

Stafford-Clark, D. and Smith, A. C. (1978) *Psychiatry of Students*, 5th edn, Allen & Unwin, London.

Stein, T. J., Gambrill, E. D. and Wiltse, K. T. (1974) 'Foster Care: The Use of Contracts', *Public Welfare*, 32, 20–25.

Stengel, E. (1973) *Suicide and Attempted Suicide*, rev. edn, Penguin, Harmondsworth.

Stern, R. S. (1978) *Behavioural Techniques*, Academic Press, London.

Stevens, B. C. (1972) 'Dependence of Schizophrenic Patients on Elderly Relatives', *Psychological Medicine*, 2, 17.

Stevens, B. C. (1973a) 'Role of Fluphenazine Decanoate in Lessening the Burden of Chronic Schizophrenics on the Community', *Psychological Medicine*, 3, 141–58.

Stevens, B. (1973b) 'Evaluation of Rehabilitation for Psychotic Patients in the Community', *Acta Psychiatry Scandinavia*, 49, 169–80.

Stewart, M. A., DeBlois, C. S. and Cummings, C. (1980) 'Psychiatric Disorder in the Parents of Hyperactive Boys and Those With Conduct Disorder', *Journal of Child Psychology and Psychiatry*, 21, 283–92.

Stöffelmayr, B. E., Faulkner, G. E. and Mitchell, W. S. (1973) 'The Rehabilitation of Chronic Hospitalised Patients: a Comparative Study of Operant Conditioning Methods and Social Therapy Techniques', *Final Report to the Scottish Home and Health Department*, London.

Storr, A. (1978) 'Sadism, Paranoia and Cruelty as a Collective and Individual Response', in Hersov, L. A., Berger, M. and Schaffer, D. (eds), *Aggression and Antisocial Behaviour in Childhood and Adolescence*, Pergamon, Oxford.

Strickler, D., Bigelow, G., Lawrence, C. and Liebson, I. (1976) 'Moderate Drinking as an Alternative to Alcohol Abuse: a Non-aversive Procedure', *Behaviour Research and Therapy*, 14, 251–67.

Strupp, H. H. and Hadley, S. W. (1979) 'Specific vs Nonspecific Factors in Psychotherapy: A Controlled Study of Outcome', *Archives of General*

Psychiatry, 36, 1125–36.

Suinn, R. M. and Richardson, F. (1971) 'Anxiety Management Training: A Nonspecific Behavior Therapy Program for Anxiety Control', *Behavior Therapy*, 2, 498–510.

Sutherland, S. (1976) *Breakdown*, Weidenfeld & Nicolson, London.

Szasz, T. S. (1974) *Law, Liberty and Psychiatry*, Routledge & Kegan Paul, London.

Taylor, Lord and Chave, S. (1964) *Mental Health and the Environment*, Longman, London.

Temerlin, M. K. (1968) 'Suggestion Effects in Psychiatric Diagnosis', *Journal of Nervous and Mental Diseases*, 147, 4, 349–53; reprinted in Scheff, T. J. (ed.), *Labeling Madness*, Prentice-Hall, 1975.

Thomas, E. J. (1977) *Marital Communication and Decision-Making*, The Free Press, New York.

Thomas, E. J. and Carter, R. D. (1971) 'Instigative Modification with a Multi Problem Family', *Social Casework*, 52, 444–55.

Tidmarsh, D. and Wood S. (1972) 'Psychiatric Aspects of Destitution', in Wing, J. K. and Hailey, A. (eds), *Evaluating a Community Psychiatric Service*, Oxford University Press, Oxford.

Toseland, R. and Rose, S. D. (1978) 'Evaluating Social Skills Training for Older Adults in Groups', *Social Work Research and Abstracts*, 1, March, 25–35.

Trower, P., Bryant, B. and Argyle, M. (1978) *Social Skills and Mental Health*, Methuen, London.

Tsuang, M. T. and VanderMey, R. (1980) *Genes and the Mind*, Oxford University Press, Oxford.

Ullman, L. P. and Krasner, L. (1975) *A Psychological Approach to Abnormal Behavior*, 2nd edn, Prentice-Hall, Englewood Cliffs, New Jersey.

Vaughn, C. E. and Leff, J. P. (1976) 'The Influence of Family and Social Factors on the Course of Psychiatric Illness', *British Journal of Psychiatry*, 129, 125–37.

Venables, P. H. (1964) 'Input Dysfunction in Schizophrenia', in Maher, B. A. (ed.), *Progress in Experimental Personality Research I*, Academic Press, New York.

Venables, P. H. (1979) 'The Psychophysiology of Schizophrenia', in Gaind, R. and Hudson, B. L. (eds), *Current Themes in Psychiatry II*, Macmillan, London.

Wallerstein, J. S. and Kelly, J. B. (1980) *Surviving the Breakup*, Grant McIntyre, London.

Wansbrough, N. (1973) 'From Psychiatric Ward to Shopfloor', *New Society*, 19 April, 128–31.

Wansbrough, N. (1980) *Sheltered Work – Open Employment*, National Schizophrenia Fellowship, Surbiton.

Wansbrough, N. and Cooper, P. (1980) *Open Employment after Mental Illness*, Tavistock, London.

Wansbrough, N., Cooper, P. and Mitchell, B. (1979) 'The Employment Patterns of Former Psychiatric Patients', in Meacher, M. (ed.), *New*

Methods of Mental Health Care, Pergamon, Oxford.

Watson, J. P. (1979) 'Psychiatric Ideologies', in Gaind, R. and Hudson, B. L. (eds), *Current Themes in Psychiatry II*, 60–8.

Watts, F. N. (1978) 'A Study of Work Behaviour in a Psychiatric Rehabilitation Unit', *British Journal of Social and Clinical Psychology*, 17, 85–92.

Weissman, M. M., Klerman, G. L., Paykel, E. S., Prusoff, B. and Hanson, B. (1974) 'Treatment Effects on the Social Adjustment of Depressed Patients', *Archives of General Psychiatry*, 30, 771–8.

Weissman, M. M., Paykel, E. S. and Klerman, G. L. (1972) 'The Depressed Woman as a Mother', *Social Psychiatry*, 7, 98–108.

Weissman, M. M., Prusoff, B. A., Dimascio, A., Neu, C., Goklaney, M. and Klerman, G. L. (1979) 'The Efficacy of Drugs and Psychotherapy in the Treatment of Acute Depressive Episodes', *American Journal of Psychiatry*, 135, 555–8.

West, D. J. and Farrington, D. P. (1973) *Who Becomes Delinquent?*, Heinemann, London.

Whiteley, J. S. (1970) 'The Response of Psychopaths to a Therapeutic Community', *British Journal of Psychiatry*, 116, 517–29.

Whiteley, J. S. (1975) 'The Psychopath and his Treatment', in Silverstone, T. and Barraclough, B. (eds), *Contemporary Psychiatry*, Royal College of Psychiatrists, London.

Whiteley, J. S., Briggs, D. and Turner, M. (1972) *Dealing with Deviants*, Hogarth, London.

Whiteley, J. S. and Gordon, J. (1979) *Group Approaches in Psychiatry*, Routledge & Kegan Paul, London.

Wild, R. (1980) 'Is AA Going Along the Right Road?', *Community Care*, 3 April, no. 309.

Wilder, J. (1978) *An Aid to Community Care*, Psychiatric Rehabilitation Association, London.

Williams, E. (1971) 'Models of Madness', *New Society*, 30 September, 607–9.

Willis, J. (1974) *Lecture Notes on Psychiatry*, 4th edn, Blackwell, Oxford.

Willis, J. (1976) *Clinical Psychiatry*, Blackwell, Oxford.

Wilson, C. (1981) 'The Impact on Children', in Orford, J. and Harwin, J. (eds), *Alcohol and the Family*, Croom Helm, London.

Windheuser, H. J. (1977) 'Anxious Mothers as Models for Coping with Anxiety', *Behavior Analysis and Therapy*, 2, 1, 39–58.

Wing, J. K. (1966) 'Social and Psychological Changes in a Rehabilitation Unit', *Social Psychiatry*, 1, 21.

Wing, J. K. (1974) 'Housing Environments and Mental Health', in Parry, H. B. (ed.), *Population and its Problems*, Oxford University Press, Oxford.

Wing, J. K. (ed.) (1975) *Schizophrenia from Within*, National Schizophrenia Fellowship, Surbiton.

Wing, J. K. (1978) *Reasoning about Madness*, Oxford University Press, Oxford.

Wing, J. K., Bennett, D. H. and Denham, J. (1964) *Industrial Rehabilitation of Long-stay Schizophrenic Patients*, Medical Research Council Memorandum No. 42, HMSO, London.

Wing, J. K. and Brown, G. (1970) *Institutionalism and Schizophrenia*, Cambridge University Press, Cambridge.

Wing, L., Wing, J. K., Stevens, B. and Griffiths, D. (1972) 'An Epidemiological and Experimental Evaluation of Industrial Rehabilitation of Chronic Psychotic Patients in the Community', in Wing, J. K. and Hailey, A. (eds), *Evaluating a Community Psychiatric Service*, Oxford University Press, Oxford.

Wolff, S. and Acton, W. P. (1968) 'Characteristics of Parents of Disturbed Children', *British Journal of Psychiatry*, 114, 593–601.

Wolpe, J. and Lazarus, A. (1966) *Behavior Therapy Techniques*, Pergamon, New York.

Woods, R. T. (1979) 'Reality Orientation and Staff Attention: A Controlled Study', *British Journal of Psychiatry*, 134, 502–7.

Wynne, L. C., Ryckoff, I., Day, J. and Hirsch, S. (1958) 'Pseudo-mutuality in the Family Relations of Schizophrenics', *Psychiatry*, 21, 205–20.

Author Index

Subject Index

Numbers in **bold face** refer to complete chapters or sections.